T0220255

Clinical Cases in Augmentative and Alternative Communication

Clinical Cases in Augmentative and Alternative Communication provides a concise introduction to the rapidly expanding field of augmentative and alternative communication (AAC). It brings together internationally renowned experts in the field to discuss its application and outline key principles of intervention to support communication using AAC.

Carefully grounded in evidence-based clinical practice, the book highlights the diversity of potential applications for AAC across a wide range of client groups, including children and adults with developmental disabilities, as well as adults with acquired impairments. Most of the chapters are structured as case reports following CARE guidelines and highlight key principles for intervention that are grounded in clinical practice. The chapters also include reflections on communication through AAC and the valuable contributions that AAC can make in supporting independence and enhancing quality of life.

This accessible book is ideal reading for students, novice clinicians in the fields of speech and language therapy or pathology, and professionals who are new to this area of clinical practice.

Martine M. Smith is Professor in Clinical Speech and Language Studies at Trinity College Dublin, Ireland. Her experience in the area of AAC stretches over three decades and is grounded in her clinical experience, research focus, and teaching. A Past President of the International Society for Augmentative and Alternative Communication and former Editor-in-Chief of the flagship journal *Augmentative and Alternative Communication* (2015–2019), she has published extensively in the field and has an international reputation as a researcher.

Clinical Cases in Speech and Language Disorders

Clinical Cases in Speech and Language Disorders is a new series of short books that each focus on a specific speech and language disorder, providing an in-depth look at real or imagined scenarios, and discussing relevant assessment and intervention plans using theory, research findings, and clinical reasoning. The overall aim of these books is to provide much-needed resources using real-life clinical cases to help clinicians and students reflect on clinical decision making involving the assessment and management of patients presenting with various speech and language disorders (SLD).

Titles in the series:

Clinical Cases in Dysarthria
Edited by Margaret Walshe and Nick Miller

Clinical Cases in Dysphagia
Edited by Margaret Walshe and Maggie-Lee Huckabee

Clinical Cases in Dysfluency
Edited by Margaret M. Leahy and Kurt Eggers

Clinical Cases in Augmentative and Alternative Communication
Edited by Martine M. Smith

For more information about this series, please visit: www.routledge.com/ Clinical-Cases-in-Speech-and-Language-Disorders/book-series/CCSLD

Clinical Cases in Augmentative and Alternative Communication

Edited by Martine M. Smith

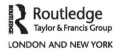
Routledge
Taylor & Francis Group

LONDON AND NEW YORK

Designed cover image: © Getty Images

First published 2023
by Routledge
4 Park Square, Milton Park, Abingdon, Oxon OX14 4RN

and by Routledge
605 Third Avenue, New York, NY 10158

Routledge is an imprint of the Taylor & Francis Group, an informa business

British Library Cataloguing-in-Publication Data
A catalogue record for this book is available from the British Library

ISBN: 978-0-367-61829-2 (hbk)
ISBN: 978-0-367-61828-5 (pbk)
ISBN: 978-1-003-10673-9 (ebk)

DOI: 10.4324/9781003106739

Typeset in Bembo
by Apex CoVantage, LLC

To Gillian, who taught me so much about parenting a child who uses AAC

Contents

Preface

Professor Martine M. Smith is an internationally renowned expert in the area of augmentative and alternative communication (AAC). Therefore, as Series Editor of *Clinical Cases in Speech and Language Disorders*, I am extremely grateful to her for leading this project as editor. With contributions from fellow clinical specialists, experts, and researchers in the field of AAC, this text on *Clinical Cases in Augmentative and Alternative Communication* promises to be another highly valuable resource for students, early career speech-language therapists or pathologists, and indeed, clinicians already working in the area of communication disorders.

In keeping with other texts in the *Clinical Cases in Speech and Language Disorders* series, this book continues to use the case report format, placing the client and family at the centre of the story that must be told. This format adds something different to the library of working clinicians and students. Despite the fact that case reports sit somewhat unfairly at the bottom of the traditional evidence pyramid, their strength lies in the fact that they reflect real life clinical contexts, expose clinical challenges, and give us valuable perspectives on clinical decision making. This is missing in traditional textbooks. Case reports can contribute to evidence for new and novel innovative approaches to client management. They can also serve to signal alarms that may exist with an established treatment. Each case report within this textbook serves to illustrate or expand on a specific clinical message or support a core theoretical argument within the field of AAC. Another valuable feature of case reports is that they allow us to hear the voices of a range of key stakeholders more readily, and multiple voices echo throughout this text.

I hope, therefore, that readers enjoy this latest offering in a series that continues to grow and develop. As well as acknowledging the work of Professor Smith, I must also thank the individual chapter authors for sharing their expertise so readily. Finally, I'd like to thank the ever-patient editorial team at Routledge for their help in bringing another highly valued contribution to the *Clinical Cases in Speech and Language Disorders* series to fruition.

Margaret Walshe
Series Editor,
Clinical Cases in Speech and Language Disorders
August 2022

Contributors

Anna A. Allen, PhD, CCC-SLP, is the Director of Clinical Care and Research at Puddingstone Place, LLC, Middleborough, MA. She has more than 15 years of clinical experience providing speech-language intervention to children with autism spectrum disorder (ASD) and other developmental disabilities. Her research focuses on the application of mobile technology to communication intervention for persons with ASD and their families.

Molly B. Allen, MS, CCC-SLP, is a speech-language pathologist at the League School of Greater Boston. She received her master's degree in speech–language pathology from MGH Institute of Health Professions in Boston, Massachusetts. Her clinical and research interests include autism spectrum disorder, and augmentative and alternative communication.

Lisa G. Bardach, MS, CCC-SLP, is a licensed, certified speech–language pathologist with more than 30 years of experience providing neurogenic rehabilitation to adult and paediatric clients. She is the owner of Communicating Solutions, a private practice in Ann Arbor, Michigan, specializing in evaluation and treatment for individuals requiring augmentative and alternative communication (AAC). She also works for ALS of Michigan, where she has developed and implemented a regional clinic to provide AAC and assistive technology (AT) services to patients with amyotrophic lateral sclerosis (ALS).

Cathy Binger, PhD, CCC-SLP, is a speech-language pathologist and professor at the University of New Mexico who specializes in AAC. Dr. Binger is an active researcher who develops and evaluates intervention programs designed to enhance the language skills of children who use AAC and valid measurements to monitor aided language progress. Her work also focuses on developing partner instruction programs – that is, programs designed to teach educators and families how to communicate more effectively with children who use AAC. Dr. Binger has coauthored several books and book chapters and has published numerous research articles in both peer-reviewed journals and clinician-oriented newsletters. She is fortunate to have longstanding collaborations with AAC researchers at the University of Central Florida, including Jennifer Kent-Walsh, Nancy Harrington, and Carolyn Buchanan.

Carolyn Buchanan, MA, CCC-SLP, ATP, CBIS, is a speech-language pathologist, assistive technology professional, and certified brain injury specialist. She is a clinical instructor at the University of Central Florida (UCF), and the regional coordinator for the Florida Alliance for Assistive Services and Technology (FAAST) Atlantic Region Demonstration Center. Ms. Buchanan teaches and presents on topics related to augmentative and alternative communication (AAC). Her clinical work is with individuals with complex communication needs across the lifespan, and she collaborates with other members of the UCF AAC Collaborative to develop AAC interventions for children who require AAC.

Nicole Choe, MS, CCC-SLP, is a speech-language pathologist in the Autism Language Program at Boston Children's Hospital. Her clinical and research interests include developing AAC tools to support receptive and expressive language development and exploring the use of available technology to support communication.

Sally Clendon, PhD, is a speech-language therapist with expertise in literacy instruction for children with complex communication and learning needs, particularly those who use augmentative and alternative communication (AAC). Sally is a Senior Lecturer in Speech and Language Therapy in the Institute of Education at Massey University in Auckland.

John Costello, MA, CCC-SLP is a speech-language pathologist with more than 35 years' experience in the area of augmentative and alternative communication at Boston Children's Hospital (BCH). He is Director of the AAC Programs at BCH and an adjunct faculty member of Boston University. Over the past three decades, he has led the field in innovations to support the preservation of self and dignity in the face of severe communication impairments and pioneered the use of message banking from the late 1990s. He has published in peer-reviewed journals and has presented widely internationally on many different aspects of AAC.

Shakila Dada, PhD, is a professor in the Centre for Augmentative and Alternative Communication (CAAC) in the Faculty of Humanities at the University of Pretoria and was recently appointed as the Director of the Centre. With her research, she seeks to systemically describe, understand, and address the communication and participation patterns of persons with complex communication needs. Her particular focus is on how graphic symbol-based augmentative and alternative communication (AAC) systems can be used to facilitate language learning for individuals with complex communication needs so as to facilitate their participation in society.

Aimee Dietz, PhD, is Professor and Department Chair at Georgia State University. She is a speech-language pathologist at heart and is dedicated to training the next generation of academic researchers and clinicians, as well as improving outcomes for people with aphasia. Her research focuses on using AAC as a language recovery tool and identifying associated neurobio-markers. In recent years, she has cultivated a new line of research that seeks to understand how mind-body practices, including adapted yoga, might be harnessed to build resilience and coping for people with post-stroke aphasia and their co-survivors.

Karen Erickson, PhD, the David E. and Dolores "Dee" Yoder Distinguished Professor in the Department of Health Sciences, School of Medicine, University of North Carolina at Chapel Hill, is the Director of the Center for Literacy and Disability Studies and a Professor in the Division of Speech and Hearing Sciences.

Gillian Fitzpatrick is a home maker and a parent of three children, one of whom, Seán, uses AAC. Gillian always believed in Seán's potential and was tireless in her pursuit of better communication access to support his participation in all aspects of life.

Seán Fitzpatrick is a young man who at the time of writing is about to embark on a new adventure in third-level education. Seán has used a wide range of aided and unaided communication systems over many years.

Suzanne Flynn, PhD, is a professor of linguistics/language acquisition and a CCC-SLP at Children's Hospital/Waltham. Her research focuses on multiple language learning in children and adults, as well as on the neural representation of the multilingual brain. She works clinically with individuals with autism spectrum disorder and focuses on research on intervention and treatment.

Maria Galassi, MS, CCC-SLP is a speech-language pathologist in the Autism Language Program at Boston Children's Hospital. She received her master's degree in speech-language pathology from MGH Institute of Health Professions in Boston, Massachusetts, and her bachelor's degree in biology from Saint Joseph's University in Philadelphia, Pennsylvania. Maria's clinical and research interests include developing innovations in AAC tools to support receptive and expressive language development.

Nancy Harrington, MA, CCC-SLP, ATP, is a speech-language pathologist, assistive technology professional, AAC Lab Research Grant Coordinator, and Associate Clinical Instructor at the University of Central Florida. Nancy has more than 35 years of clinical and research experience in the United States and Ireland, with a focus on individuals with complex communication needs.

Jennifer Kent-Walsh, PhD, CCC-SLP, ASHA Fellow, is Professor of Communication Sciences and Disorders, Director of the FAAST Assistive Technology Center, and Associate Dean of Research in the College of Health Professions and Sciences at the University of Central Florida. Dr. Kent-Walsh and her research collaborators develop and evaluate interventions designed to improve language and communication outcomes for children who use AAC.

Michelle Kryc is a practicing speech-language pathologist in Denver, Colorado. She works in both inpatient and outpatient rehabilitation. She specializes in working with individuals with neurogenic communication disorders and has an interest in augmentative and alternative communication.

Yvonne Lynch, PhD, is a speech and language therapist and lecturer at Trinity College Dublin. She teaches at the undergraduate and postgraduate levels and her research interests include augmentative and alternative communication (AAC), language interventions, telepractice, and clinical decision making.

Adele May is a speech and language therapist who completed her undergraduate degree in 2004. She has garnered clinical skills for assessment and management in persons with a wide range of disabilities. She developed an interest in designing participation-based interventions for persons with communication disability during her master's degree at the Center for Augmentative and Alternative Communication (CAAC), at the University of Pretoria, South Africa. She completed her PhD in AAC under the supervision of Prof. Shakila Dada and Prof. Janice Murray. Her niche research interest is AAC in persons with dementia; specifically, AAC that is person centred, evidence based, and participatory in design.

Muireann McCleary is a speech and language therapist with extensive clinical experience working with children and adults with significant disabilities. Her key clinical and research interests include language and interaction in aided communication, as well as family-centred assessment and intervention practices. She is currently Speech and Language Therapy Manager at the Central Remedial Clinic in Dublin, Ireland.

Loren F. McMahon, OTD, OTR/L, is an occupational therapist within the Augmentative Communication Program at Boston Children's Hospital. Loren received her doctorate from MGH Institute of Health Professions, where she focused on assistive technology through collaboration with the Open Style Lab at the Massachusetts Institute of Technology. In practice, Loren provides solutions for alternative access, mounting, seating and positioning, and environmental controls for adults and children with complex motor and communication needs. She has presented nationally and internationally at the American Occupational Therapy Association (AOTA), the American Speech-Language-Hearing Association (ASHA), Assistive Technology Industry Association (ATIA), The Boston Museum of Science, the Massachusetts Association for Occupational Therapy (MAOT), RESNA, and the World Federation of Occupational Therapists (WFOT).

Janice Murray, PhD, is a professor in the Faculty of Health and Education at Manchester Metropolitan University. Her research interests include language development through aided means and how aided language learning supports educational attainment, inclusion, and participatory opportunity for those with complex communication needs. She is particularly interested in the communication aid identification and recommendation process.

Ralf W. Schlosser holds a PhD in severe disabilities and augmentative and alternative communication (AAC) from Purdue University. He is a professor in the Departments of Communication Sciences and Disorders and Applied Psychology at Northeastern University and the Director of Clinical Research at the Center for Communication Enhancement at Boston Children's Hospital. Ralf has published extensively on AAC interventions for children with developmental disabilities, including studies, systematic reviews, and books. He is a fellow of the American Association on Intellectual and Developmental Disabilities (AAIDD), the American Speech-Language-Hearing Association (ASHA), and the International Society for Augmentative and Alternative Communication (ISAAC).

Howard C. Shane, PhD, is the Director of the Center for Communication Enhancement at Boston Children's Hospital. He is an associate professor at Harvard Medical School, and Professor of Communication Sciences and Disorders at MGH Institute for Health Professions. He is a fellow of the American Speech-Language-Hearing Association (ASHA) and a recipient of their Honors of the Association award. He is the author of numerous research papers, chapters, and books on severe speech impairment and has lectured throughout the world on the topic.

Martine M. Smith, PhD, is a speech and language therapist and professor in Clinical Speech and Language Studies at Trinity College Dublin. Her research focuses on language and literacy learning in the context of augmentative and alternative communication (AAC), as well as the impact of AAC on interaction and participation.

Leigh Anne White, MEd, MS, CCC-SLP, is a speech-language pathologist in the Autism Language Program within the Center for Communication Enhancement at Boston Children's Hospital. Her research interests include autism spectrum disorder, augmentative and alternative communication, and play-based language interventions. Leigh Anne received her master's degree in education with a concentration in human development and psychology from Harvard University and her master's degree in speech-language pathology from Boston University.

Christina Yu, MS, CCC-SLP, is a speech-language pathologist in the Autism Language Program and Augmentative Communication Program at Boston Children's Hospital. Her research interests include exploring the use of available technology to support communication, factors in augmentative and alternative communication (AAC) assessment outcomes, and the creation of developmentally based assessment and interventions for individuals who use AAC.

1 Introduction to Clinical Cases in Augmentative and Alternative Communication (AAC)

Martine M. Smith

The field of augmentative and alternative communication (AAC) has transformed over the roughly six decades since the term was first coined (Zangari et al., 1994), not only in the tools, resources, and strategies that are employed, but also in terms of target client groups, models for decision making and expectations of outcomes. These changes have occurred against a backdrop of fundamental paradigm shifts in models of ability and disability, transformation of the role of evidence-based decision making within interventions and technological innovations. However, some fundamentals remain the same. Clinicians and practitioners need to build relationships with families, individual clients, and other key stakeholders to understand the communication needs and opportunities that are available. They also need to build collaborative goals so that investment on the part of the client and their families results in meaningful and impactful change in social participation, autonomy, and self-fulfilment. This text provides an introduction to the application of AAC across a wide range of client groups, including children and adults with developmental disabilities (e.g., Chapters 3–7), as well as adults with acquired impairments (Chapters 9–12). Most chapters are structured around a case report, so that the principles that underpin intervention are illustrated using examples that are grounded in clinical practice. Chapter 2 is not a traditional case report; instead, it illustrates the application of an approach to AAC clinical decision making with reference to a school-aged student. Chapter 8 represents a very personal account, as a parent and her adult son reflect on their communication journey in a powerful illustration of the vital role and contribution that AAC can make in enhancing quality of life and maintaining personhood. Collectively, the chapters included here illustrate some key points in relation to AAC: the diversity of potential applications, the different roles and purposes it can serve, as well as the importance of creative clinicians and resilient clients and stakeholders in ensuring that the potential benefits AAC can offer are exploited to best effect.

The rest of this chapter revisits some core principles of intervention with individuals with communication impairments, explores concepts and terminology that are commonly used in relation to AAC and outlines key principles underpinning intervention using AAC, which are illustrated in the many

DOI: 10.4324/9781003106739-1

chapters that follow. Finally, this chapter provides an overview of the issues illustrated in the case reports in subsequent chapters.

Grounding Intervention in Evidence-Based Practice

Although clinical practice has always sought to bring about measurable change based on rigorous observation of the impact of intervention on individual clients, the rise of the conceptual framework of evidence-based practice (EBP) has reshaped expectations of how clinical decisions are guided and rationalised. Since its inception, it has been widely accepted that EBP requires the integration of at least three sources of information: "the best external evidence with individual clinical expertise and patients' choice" (Sackett et al., 1996, p. 72). Few would argue with the merits of basing clinical decisions on the best available evidence, but controversies continue about what constitutes evidence, and how different kinds of evidence should be valued (e.g., Archibald, 2015; Kovarsky & Curran, 2007). Despite these controversies, the EBP movement has reshaped expectations of what kind of information is important to consider when working with clients to enhance their communication. It has formalised the requirement to explicitly consider the knowledge that is relevant to the field, the information that we learn about a client in every interaction, whether direct or indirect, and the unique experiences, concerns, and aspirations of that client, to build interventions that make a meaningful difference. One challenge in AAC is staying abreast of current knowledge, given the rapid developments in technology for communication devices and in the ways those technologies can be accessed. The pace of these developments can raise concerns that any device recommended is outdated by the time it is delivered. However, waiting for the perfect solution is not an option – the loss of time and opportunity for learning is more significant than any perceived loss of efficiency of a device. No device will ever be perfect and every device costs time to learn.

AAC has tended to be a practice-led field (von Tetzchner & Grove, 2003b), partly because of this rapid technological change that is out of synch with the normal rhythms of research and publication. Expert clinicians, manufacturers, and distributors serve important functions as sources of knowledge, but reliance on these sources puts an even greater onus on individual clinicians to be grounded in sound principles of assessment and intervention and to critically interrogate evidence to arrive at solutions that are principled, problem focused, and informed. As pointed out by Sackett et al. (1996), evidence does not make decisions, people do.

The right to freedom of expression of opinion has been enshrined as an internationally recognised fundamental human right for more than 70 years, in Article 19 of the Universal Declaration of Human Rights (United Nations, 1948). Almost 60 years later, this fundamental right was further specified in Article 21 of the Convention on the Rights of Persons with Disabilities (United Nations, 2006) to include the right of individuals to "seek, receive and impart information and ideas on an equal basis with others and through all forms of communication of their choice", including through the use of augmentative and alternative communication. The Communication Bill of Rights (Brady et al., 2016) asserts 15 fundamental communication rights, including the right to always have access to functioning AAC, and the right to have clear, meaningful, and culturally and linguistically appropriate communication. Specifying that access to AAC is a right highlights the importance of AAC in enabling individuals with significant impairments to claim their role within society.

Terminology in Augmentative and Alternative Communication

As with any field of practice, some terminology has evolved that is specifically relevant to AAC. The term *augmentative and alternative communication* itself highlights potentially important distinctions in the role that nonspeech modalities may play in supporting communication. Some individuals can produce speech or vocalisations that are intelligible to some communication partners at least some of the time, but they require augmentation of those speech-production abilities for other situations. Other individuals can produce little if any speech and rely on nonspeech modalities in almost all situations. Because natural speech is such a powerful and pervasive form of communication, the distinction between systems that augment existing speech abilities versus those that serve as an alternative to speech production can be important in terms of expectations, acceptance, and motivation for all involved. It is worth noting that the use of natural sign languages (e.g., Irish Sign Language, British Sign Language) as a first (or second) language does not come under the term AAC, as these are full natural languages, comparable to any spoken language.

Nonspeech modalities are typically categorised as either *unaided* or *aided*. Unaided modes rely on the physical resources of the individual speaker, and include modes such as gestures, manual sign, facial expression, vocalizations, body movements, and eye gaze. Aided modes involve using something external to the speaker. External aids can be simple, involving no technology (i.e., *no tech*), such as a pen, a paper-based alphabet, or symbol communication board or book. Some *low tech* or *light tech* aided modes utilise simple technologies, such as battery-operated devices that can record a small number of messages (e.g., a BIGmack™). *High tech* aided modes use some form of computer technology and typically incorporate the potential for voice output. These include *dedicated* devices developed specifically as communication aids, as well as mainstream platforms, such as laptops or tablet technologies, onto which specific software is loaded. Terms commonly used to refer to this last group include *voice output communication aids* (VOCAs) and *speech-generating devices* (SGDs).

Regardless of the type of communication aid, the language that is to be used to communicate with others must be represented on that aid. The most widely used *representational form* is written language, whether alphabetically or morphologically based (i.e., letters or words). Many individuals who need to use aided communication do not have the skills needed to rely on written language and so alternative representational systems are necessary, most often in the form of graphic symbols that can range from photos through to abstract symbol systems (see Beukelman and Mirenda (2013) for a comprehensive description of types of symbols). Regardless of the potential power of a particular communication aid, unless the language representational system is appropriate to the individual user, it is unlikely that it will support communication effectively.

A final term relates to *access methods* – how an individual selects the individual letter, symbol, or message that is to be communicated. Using *direct access* an individual can directly point to or otherwise indicate or select the target symbol (e.g., using eye gaze technologies). Many individuals who need to use aided communication do not have the physical control to efficiently point to small cells on a communication board or a screen; instead, they rely on *indirect access*. Sometimes indirect access involves getting assistance from a communication partner, who scans letters or symbols until the aided communicator indicates that the target symbol has been reached. If a high-tech system is used, a wide range of switches can be attached to the device, so that the user can select the target symbol by activating the switch. Identifying the most effective and efficient access method is an important step in facilitating the use of aided communication (Murray et al., 2019) and requires input from a wide range of disciplines.

Principles of Intervention in Augmentative and Alternative Communication

1. *AAC is an umbrella term covering a wide diversity of tools, strategies, and purposes:* AAC strategies may serve a relatively small role in the overall communication toolkit of any given individual, or may represent core, essential supports for both comprehension and expression. The purpose may be to maximise the functionality of existing speech skills (e.g., Chapter 11), to support the retention of interaction skills (see Chapter 12) or to facilitate the development of new skills (e.g., see Chapters 3–7). The limits of the application of AAC are ultimately down to the creativity of individual clinicians, educators, and family members. At the same time, there are important distinctions between completely relying on AAC to understand and participate in the world, and using some aided strategies to enhance speech intelligibility in clearly defined contexts or with specific communication partners (von Tetzchner & Martinsen, 2000). The learning needs, motivation, and expectations of what AAC might deliver in these two scenarios are very different. If someone expects to use AAC only for a short period of time (e.g., in an intensive care hospital environment), then learning demands should be minimal, so that all effort can go into communicating. By contrast, if AAC is expected to be a critical developmental support that will evolve into a comprehensive system to

support language, literacy, and social interaction, then it is worth investing significant time to learn the skills, strategies, and supports that will
maximize its potential.

2. *AAC must be integrated into a total multimodal communication system:*
All communicators use multiple modes to enhance their communicative
effectiveness. The organisation and coordination of multiple modes is
complex (Cravotta et al., 2019; Smith, 1997), and relatively little research
has focused on how children learn to combine modes effectively (but
see Heim & Baker-Mills, 1996). For even the most expert communicators, aided communication is only one option within an array of communication modes that include facial expression, speech or vocalisation,
gesture, body movements, and eye gaze (Rackensperger et al., 2005;
Smith & Connolly, 2008). The responsibility of professionals working
with individuals who might benefit from AAC is to ensure that they
facilitate the development of robust, integrated multimodal communication systems that include natural speech or vocalisations alongside other
unaided and aided modalities. True competence is characterised by being
able to choose to use aided communication when it is most likely to
enhance communicative success. One intervention challenge is ensuring
that individual clients have sufficient opportunity to become skilled in
using AAC across contexts so that they are in a good position to make
informed choices about using aided communication (Smith & Murray,
2011).

3. *Proactive engagement is important to ensure access to communication as
a fundamental human right:* Ensuring that individuals who could benefit
from aided and/or unaided modes of communication have access to appropriate access to those resources is a key responsibility of all those who support individuals with communication impairments, regardless of the extent
of their disabilities (Brady et al., 2016). One of the more persistent myths
about AAC is the concern that introducing manual signs, graphic symbols,
or voice output devices might interfere with natural speech, despite longstanding evidence that access to voice output does not inhibit and may even
promote speech production (Millar et al., 2006; Schlosser & Wendt, 2008).
Individuals whose use of AAC fits in the supportive category suggested by
von Tetzchner and Martinsen (2000), often leave AAC options behind as
their access to natural speech increases (see the case of Dean in Chapter 3).
Adopting a 'wait and see' approach to introducing AAC positions these
modes as a sign of failure (to develop speech or loss of speech) and deprives
individuals of vital learning opportunities, often at the most critical stages
of development.

4. *Identifying the most appropriate AAC system is an ongoing dynamic process:*
This requires consideration of at least three areas: the client, the context (including communication partners), and the communication message or content. The framework of the International Classification of

Functioning, Disability and Health (ICF; World Health Organization, 2001) provides a robust structure to guide assessment, ensuring that communication opportunities, needs, barriers, and facilitators (Beukelman & Mirenda, 2013) are front and centre in information gathering, to maximize the potential impact of any intervention. Over time, communication needs change, as do physical abilities, technology potentials, and language and learning resources (e.g., see Chapters 7 and 10). For this reason, AAC systems are always a work in progress. It is important that there is a clear pathway to support individuals and families to update, revise, extend, or change components within those systems.

5. ***Development implies change, both planned and unplanned:*** Beukelman and Mirenda (1992, 2013) highlighted the importance of planning not only for today, but also for tomorrow. Tomorrows are unpredictable. As many of the cases described in this text illustrate, developmental changes open new opportunities, but also new learning challenges. When engaging with a young preschool child for whom communication is difficult, it is impossible to predict where exactly development might lead. Intervention must be planned in stages, in sequences of steps that are manageable. Explicitly considering how well individual steps in intervention feed into long-term goals of supporting relationships, independence, and self-fulfilment helps to ensure that the ultimate outcome is of meaningful value to that individual and their family (Smith & Murray, 2011). For most children, learning the language of their community is an unplanned (albeit finely tuned) process, embedded in rich social interactions. By contrast, learning to use AAC, whether aided or unaided, typically occurs within planned, structured interventions, often directed by someone who, at least initially, is unfamiliar with either the child or the family (von Tetzchner, 2018; von Tetzchner & Grove, 2003a). The outcomes of an immersive language learning experience are predictable – competence in the language of the community. The outcomes arising from AAC interventions are less clear, with no definitive developmental map (Smith, 2015) and influenced by a host of additional factors, both intrinsic to the individual using AAC and external factors within the environment that come into play.

6. ***An alternative AAC: Adversity, Adaptability, and Creativity (Smith, 2017):*** Learning to use AAC takes time and effort. Interacting using modes of communication that are atypical, or at least less common, makes it more difficult for everyone in the interaction to achieve mutual understanding. Aided communication is slow, relative to spoken language, even for skilled users, and takes considerably more effort (Light & McNaughton, 2014; Janice Murray & Goldbart, 2011; Stadskleiv et al., 2014). Communication breakdown is not uncommon (von Tetzchner, 2015) and communication partners may compensate by assuming responsibility for the structure and topic of conversations (Clarke & Kirton, 2003; Smith et al., 2016).

Individuals who use aided communication must develop the resilience needed to cope with these interaction adversities. They must accommodate to a constantly changing technological world, where familiar systems are updated or discontinued (Smith, 2019) in time frames over which they have no control. To overcome communication breakdown, they and their communication partners must be creative as well as resilient, solving communication problems by drawing on multiple resources (Neuvonen et al., 2022).

7. *Communicative competence is multilayered and dynamic:* Light's model of communicative competence (1989; Light & McNaughton, 2014) set out four domains of competence to consider in unaided and particularly aided communication: linguistic, social, strategic, and operational. These domains provide a valuable point of reference for assessment and intervention. Communicative competence is neither static nor solely owned by any one individual. It is constructed in the moment of interaction, influenced by each participant in an interaction, as well as by the demands or challenges of the communication content and context. Even highly skilled communicators can feel incompetent if they must communicate information that is outside their area of expertise, or in an unfamiliar or challenging context. Individuals who use AAC can be remarkably successful in interactions with some communication partners, and yet struggle to achieve any mutual understanding with other partners, even though their own skills and resources have not changed. Enhancing communicative competence implies considering both the individual using AAC and also those with whom they interact.

8. *Communication should not be hard work, even if sometimes it is a hard-won prize:* Aided communication requires far more effort, both physically and cognitively, than using natural speech. It also takes longer. Individuals need opportunities to become proficient in operational skills (i.e., in using their system) without the pressure of immediate communication demands. They need access to language learning opportunities, in contexts where other demands are minimal, as discussed in Chapter 4. Their attempts at communication need to be recognised, acknowledged, and supported so that they learn the potential power of communication, power that can motivate them to persist and become proficient in the wide range of skills essential to effective use of AAC. Many children and adults who use aided communication experience challenges in all aspects of their lives. Opportunities for laughter and leisure are just as important as therapy interventions in terms of quality of life (King et al., 2014; Zijlstra & Vlaskamp, 2015), and can be even more demanding on parents and families (Hajjar et al., 2016). Being mindful of these competing demands and priorities is important in building meaningful interventions that address authentically important goals that enhance quality of life.

9. ***Building language for communication encompasses spoken, written, signed, and graphic forms:*** Becoming a competent speller unlocks potentially unlimited vocabulary for individuals who rely on aided communication. Developing literacy skills has pervasive benefits in terms of leisure, learning, and vocational opportunities, as well as interaction across time and space through social media platforms. For individuals for whom horizons might otherwise be limited by physical or cognitive impairments, literacy skills can significantly enhance participation in society (Caron & Light, 2016; Hynan et al., 2015). However, there is longstanding evidence that many individuals who could benefit from aided communication struggle to achieve functional literacy skills, even when other areas of skill development suggest they should be able to learn to read and write (Smith, 2005). As outlined in Chapter 5, supporting literacy development requires consideration of aided language, spoken language, and written language affordances and demands. Although the learning demands on individuals who use aided communication are often greater because of the range of difficulties they experience, it is essential to ensure that support for literacy skills is positioned as one dimension of their fundamental right to access to communication.

10. ***Communicative competence is a means to an end:*** Ultimately the goal of interventions for individuals who need to use AAC is to build independence, autonomy, and inclusion. Autonomy and independence imply the freedom to make what might be perceived by others as 'bad' choices – including a choice not to use AAC. Our role as interventionists is to ensure those choices are informed (see for example Chapter 11), and that doors remain open for individuals and their families to return and revisit earlier decisions (as detailed in Chapter 10).

The nine case reports in this volume illustrate the application of these principles across client groups as diverse as young children with a diagnosis of autism spectrum disorder (Chapters 6 and 7) to older adults facing a neurodegenerative disease (Chapter 11) or dementia (Chapter 12). Chapters 3 and 4 describe the unpredictability that often surrounds the introduction of aided communication with young children whose developmental trajectory is always uncertain. Chapter 5 reviews the critical importance of integrated, multidimensional interventions to effectively enhance literacy learning. Chapters 6 and 7 outline the value of systematic, data-based assessment and intervention for young children with a diagnosis of autism spectrum disorder, to support all aspects of their communication development. In Chapter 9, the potential benefits of AAC for individuals with aphasia is outlined, recognising that it may play a discrete but nonetheless important role in supporting interaction and participation. Chapter 10 reviews a 20-year journey with AAC with Kay, who sustained a severe traumatic brain injury when she was 18 years old. In Chapter 11, the case of Andrew is presented, detailing his challenges as he faced a diagnosis of motor neurone disease and the valuable role AAC played in sustaining his identity and role within the family. Chapter 12 presents Elizabeth, whose use of AAC was relatively brief, but for whom it enabled her family and her caregivers to continue to include her in positive social interactions and to assert her unique personality and life history as she navigated the challenge of dementia. Individually and collectively these case reports highlight the valuable role that AAC can play in supporting independence, autonomy, and inclusion.

References

Archibald, T. (2015). "They just know": The epistemological politics of "evidence-based" non-formal education. *Evaluation and Program Planning, 48*, 137–148. doi:10.1016/j.evalprogplan.2014.08.0010149-7189

Beukelman, D. R., & Mirenda, P. (1992). *Augmentative and alternative communication: Management of severe communication disorders in children and adults.* Paul H. Brooks.

Beukelman, D. R., & Mirenda, P. (2013). *Augmentative and alternative communication: Support children and adults with complex communication needs* (4th ed.). Brookes Publishing.

Brady, N., Bruce, S., Goldman, A., Erikson, K., Mineo, B., Ogletree, B., . . . Wilkinson, K. (2016). Communication services and supports for individuals with severe disabilities: Guidance for assessment and intervention. *American Journal on Intellectual and Developmental Disabilities, 121*(2), 121–138. doi:10.1352/1944-7558-121.2.121

Caron, J., & Light, J. (2016). Social media experiences of adolescents and young adults with cerebral palsy who use augmentative and alternative communication. *International Journal of Speech-Language Pathology, 19*(1), 30–42. doi:10.3109/17549507.2016.1143970

Clarke, M., & Kirton, A. (2003). Patterns of interaction between children with physical disabilities using augmentative and alternative communication and their peers. *Child Language Teaching and Therapy, 19*(2), 135–151.

Cravotta, A., Busá, M. G., & Prieto, P. (2019). Effects of encouraging the use of gestures on speech. *Journal of Speech, Language, and Hearing Research, 62*, 3204–3219. doi:10.1044/2019_JSLHR-S-18-0493

Hajjar, D., McCarthy, J., Beningno, J., & Chabot, J. (2016). "You get more than you give": Experiences of community partners in facilitating active recreation with individuals who have complex communication needs. *Augmentative and Alternative Communication, 32*(2), 131–142.

Heim, M., & Baker-Mills, A. (1996). Early development of symbolic communication and linguistic complexity through augmentative and alternative communication. In S. von Tetzchner & M. Jensen (Eds.), *Augmentative and alternative communication: European perspectives* (pp. 232–248). Whurr.

Hynan, A., Goldbart, J., & Murray, J. (2015). A grounded theory of Internet and social media use by young people who use augmentative and alternative communication (AAC). *Disability and Rehabilitation, 37*(17), 1559–1575. doi:10.3109/09638288.2015.1056387

King, G., Gibson, B., Mistry, B., Pinto, M., Goh, F., Teachman, G., . . . Thompson, L. (2014). An integrated methods study of the experiences of youth with severe disabilities in leisure activity settings: The importance of belonging, fun and control and choice. *Disability and Rehabilitation, 36*(19), 1626. doi:10.3109/09638288.2013.863389

Kovarsky, D., & Curran, M. (2007). A missing voice in the discourse of evidence-based practice. *Topics in Language Disorders, 27*, 50–61.

Light, J. (1989). Toward a definition of communicative competence for individuals using augmentative and alternative communication systems. *Augmentative and Alternative Communication, 5*, 137–144.

Light, J., & McNaughton, D. (2014). Communicative competence for individuals who require augmentative and alternative communication: A new definition for a new era of communication? *Augmentative and Alternative Communication, 30*(1), 1–18.

Millar, D., Light, J., & Schlosser, R. (2006). The impact of augmentative and alternative communication intervention on the speech production of individuals with developmental disabilities: A research review. *Journal of Speech, Language and Hearing Research, 49*, 248–264. doi:1092-4388/06/4902-0248

Murray, J., & Goldbart, J. (2011). Emergence of working memory in children using aided communication. *Journal of Assistive Technologies, 5*, 214–232. doi:10.1108/17549451111190623

Murray, J., Lynch, Y., Meredith, S., Moulam, L., Goldbart, J., Smith, M., . . . Judge, S. (2019). Professionals' decision-making in recommending communication aids in the UK: Competing considerations. *Augmentative and Alternative Communication, 35*(3), 167–179. doi:10.1080/07434618.2019.1597384

Neuvonen, K., Launonen, K., Smith, M., Stadskleiv, K., & von Tetzchner, S. (2022). Strategies in conveying information about unshared events using aided communication. *Child Language Teaching and Therapy, 38*(1), 78–94. doi:10.1177/02656590211050865

Rackensperger, T., Krezman, C., McNaughton, D., Williams, M. B., & D'Silva, K. (2005). "When I first got it, I wanted to throw it off a cliff": The challenges and benefits of learning AAC technologies as described by adults who use AAC. *Augmentative and Alternative Communication, 21*(3), 165–186.

Sackett, D., Rosenberg, W. M., Gray, J., Haynes, R. B., & Richardson, W. S. (1996). Evidence based medicine: What it is and what it isn't. *British Medical Journal, 312*, 71–72.

Schlosser, R., & Wendt, O. (2008). Effects of augmentative and alternative communication intervention on speech production in children with autism: A systematic review. *American Journal of Speech Language Pathology, 17*, 212–230. doi:1058-0360/08/1703-0212

Smith, M. (1997). The bi-modal situation of children developing alternative modes of language. In E. Björck-Akesson & P. Lindsay (Eds.), *Communication . . . naturally* (pp. 12–18). Mälardalen University Press.

Smith, M. (2005). *Literacy and augmentative and alternative communication*. Elsevier Academic Press.

Smith, M. (2015). Language development of individuals who required aided communication: Reflections on state of the science and future research directions. *Augmentative and Alternative Communication, 31*(3), 215–233. doi:10.3109/07434618.2015.1062553

Smith, M. (2017). *AAC, creativity and challenges: Unpicking an acronym*. Paper presented at the Symposium in honour of Prof Stephen von Tetzchner.

Smith, M. (2019). Innovations for supporting communication: Opportunities and challenges for people with complex communication needs. *Folia Phoniatrica et Logopedia, 71*, 156–167. doi:10.1159/000496729

Smith, M., & Connolly, I. (2008). Roles of aided communication: Perspectives of adults who use AAC. *Disability and Rehabilitation: Assistive Technology, 3*(5), 260–273. doi:10.1080/17483100802338499

Smith, M., McCague, E., O'Gara, J., & Sammon, S. (2016). Naturally speaking adults using aided communication. In M. Smith & J. Murray (Eds.), *The silent partner: Language, interaction and aided communication* (pp. 269–287). J&R Press.

Smith, M., & Murray, J. (2011). Parachute without a ripcord: The skydive of communication interaction. *Augmentative and Alternative Communication, 27*(4), 292–303. doi:10.310 9/07434618.2011.630022

Stadskleiv, K., von Tetzchner, S., Batorowicz, B., van Balkom, H., Dahlgren-Sandberg, A., & Renner, G. (2014). Investigating executive functions in children with severe speech and movement disorders using structured tasks. *Frontiers in Psychology, 5*(Article 992), 1–14. doi:10.3389/fpsyg.2014.00992

United Nations. (1948). *Universal declaration of human rights.* www.un.org/en/about-us/universal-declaration-of-human-rights

United Nations. (2006). *Convention on the rights of persons with disabilities.* www.un.org/development/desa/disabilities/convention-on-the-rights-of-persons-with-disabilities.html

von Tetzchner, S. (2015). The semiotics of aided language development. *Cognitive Development, 26,* 180–190. doi:10.1016/j.cogdev.2015.09.009

von Tetzchner, S. (2018). Introduction to the special issue on aided language processes, development, and use: An international perspective. *Augmentative and Alternative Communication, 34*(1), 1–15. doi:10.1080/07434618.2017.1422020

von Tetzchner, S., & Grove, N. (2003a). *Augmentative and alternative communication: Developmental issues.* Whurr.

von Tetzchner, S., & Grove, N. (2003b). The development of alternative language forms. In S. von Tetzchner & N. Grove (Eds.), *Augmentative and alternative communication: Developmental issues* (pp. 1–27). Whurr.

von Tetzchner, S., & Martinsen, H. (2000). *Introduction to augmentative and alternative communication* (2nd ed.). Whurr.

World Health Organization. (2001). *International classification of functioning, disability and health.* World Health Organisation.

Zangari, C., Lloyd, L., & Vicker, B. (1994). Augmentative and alternative communication: An historic perspective. *Augmentative and Alternative Communication, 10*(1), 27–59.

Zijlstra, H. P., & Vlaskamp, C. (2015). Leisure provision for persons with profound intellectual and multiple disabilities: Quality time or killing time? *Journal of Intellectual Disability Research, 9,* 434–448.

2 The I-ASC Explanatory Model as a Support for AAC Assessment Planning

A Case Report

Yvonne Lynch and Janice Murray

Application of the I-ASC Explanatory Model as a Support for AAC Assessment Planning

Introduction

Choosing the best possible communication aid for a child or young person is a complex process potentially involving many people who must consider multiple factors (Beukelman & Mirenda, 2013), including what symbols to use, what vocabulary is available, the preferred method of physical access, cost, portability, acceptability, and many other aid attributes. As a result, the decision-making process is highly individualised for each child and family. Decision aids help people participate in decision making about personal health care options (http://ipdas.ohri.ca/what.html). In this chapter, we present a decision aid that can support evidence-based decision making in AAC.

The tool was developed through a funded three-year National Institute for Health Research (NIHR) project (Health Services & Delivery Research Project: 14/70/153, *Identifying Appropriate Symbol Communication aids for children who are non-speaking: Enhancing clinical decision making* (I-ASC, *pronounced 'I ask'*). Findings from the project were synthesised and used to develop the I-ASC explanatory model of clinical decision making in AAC. The model provides a way of using the research findings to support critical thinking about decisions related to choosing communication aids. The model (Figure 2.1) provides a schematic representation of the complexity of the decision-making process. This chapter will illustrate the model with case data to demonstrate how it can structure thinking and inform AAC assessment and decision-making processes.

Overview of the I-ASC Explanatory Model of AAC Decision Making

The model, a theoretical conceptualisation developed from a synthesis of research data, depicts factors that influence decisions about which communication system to choose for a child or young person and how it will be

DOI: 10.4324/9781003106739-2

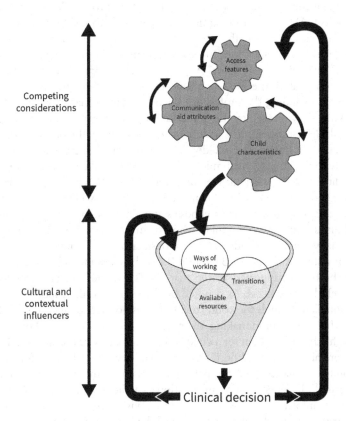

Figure 2.1 The I-ASC explanatory model of AAC decision making. Reproduced from Murray et al. (2020).

supported. The top half of the model describes the competing considerations, or the trade-offs between child characteristics, access features, and communication aid attributes. As information in one cog is considered, it may cause a shift in another cog, changing the likely preferred aid recommendation options. For example, an initial focus might be on the child's skills and abilities. If assessment indicates that a child has strong linguistic skills, communication ability, and emerging literacy skills, attention might shift to the range of communication aids that will provide the child with robust language packages through graphic symbols. Taking the child's motor abilities into account, it may be clear that the aid must also be light enough to carry when they walk. Immediately, a different set of communication aid options are needed to meet both the portability and linguistic criteria.

The purpose of decision making at this stage is to ensure the highest priorities for the child and family are met, and the communication aid is the best fit possible. This process of finding the best fit is often referred to as feature matching (Beukelman & Mirenda, 2013). Feature matching constitutes one aspect of the assessment and recommendation process (Van Niekerk et al., 2017). The I-ASC model recognises the need to choose the best fit possible, based on a series of trade-offs rather than perfect options (Murray et al., 2019). Once a decision is made about these factors, further issues external to the child or the aid can influence the final AAC recommendation (Lynch et al., 2019).

The second half of the model captures the factors related to the child's culture and context, including the professionals' work setting(s) that may influence decision making. As visualised by the funnel and its contents (ways of working, transitions, available resources), these cultural and contextual influencers denote factors that influence clinical decision making outside the competing considerations linked specifically to the child. A team might identify a potential best fit based on a child's skills, abilities, needs, and available communication aids. This tentative decision is then filtered through the cultural context where the aid will be implemented. For example, a team might decide to choose system A as the best fit for linguistic and other abilities. However, the child's school is much more familiar with system B and has many children already using it. Considering this context, the team might shift from system A to system B. System B may be a less ideal choice for the child, but may be better supported within that child's environment and therefore ultimately yield better success. As denoted by the arrows on the model, the decision that is funnelled through the contextual factors is not necessarily the final decision or the end of the decision making; the process is fluid and iterative. For example, a team might choose a system for a child and arrange a trial of that system. The team learns more about the child on the system trial, how the aid works for them, and their context. What seemed the perfect choice may emerge as presenting many unanticipated challenges. New information can cause a shift in how the model components inform decisions, resulting in a revised system-trial decision. In this way, priorities are sifted and confirmed until the best match is determined.

Recognising the complexity of the decision-making process, a range of evidence-based resources were developed to support the use of the I-ASC model in making clinical decisions. These resources support specific groups (e.g., children, families, professionals) or target distinct decision-making stages (e.g., first AAC appointment, review appointment). The I-ASC explanatory model and associated resources are freely available online (https://iasc.mmu.ac.uk/). In this chapter, we illustrate how the model and related resources can be used to plan assessments for children and young people, using the case of Gita, aged 9.

Step 1. Gather Information to Plan AAC Assessment

A critical first step in any AAC assessment involves gathering, synthesising, and prioritising information. A lack of information gathering or sharing can impact decision making (Lynch et al., 2019), potentially negatively affecting future outcomes, and so the time taken to gather and consider all relevant information before the assessment is essential. Often AAC assessments begin with a referral letter like the one shown in Figure 2.2.

This initial referral letter does not indicate which aspects of information are most relevant or influential to the AAC decision-making process for Gita.

Speech & Language Therapy Service
The Clinic, 1b, Tyndale Street, Manchester, UK

Dear Speech and Language Therapist,

I would like to refer the following child to you for an AAC assessment. Gita is 9 years and two months old. Gita has cerebral palsy and a hearing impairment, corrected with bilateral hearing aids. She effectively uses her own powered wheelchair. She can say a few words, her gag reflex is intact, and she has been prescribed patches for drooling.

She lives at home with Mum, Dad, Grandma, her 13-year-old sister, Smita, and 5-year-old brother, Jamal. Gita and Jamal both attend St Mark's special school.

Gita is reported to be doing well at school. She has a picture book to help communication and accesses hydrotherapy onsite. Gita's teacher reports that she switches off in class at times and can be hard to engage in schoolwork.

I would appreciate if you could assess Gita to see if she would benefit from any further speech and language therapy supports,

Yours sincerely,
Dr Scott
Paediatrician

Figure 2.2 Gita's referral letter

Consequently, more information about Gita was needed to plan the assessment.

Jamie, the local speech and language therapist (SLT), continued Gita's referral process with a phone call to her mother, Aesha. Aesha described Gita's homelife in the centre of a large city, where Gita enjoys playing in their garden with her brother Jamal. Gita shares a ground floor bedroom with her Grandma. Gita loves animals and her cat, Fluffy. She adores LOL dolls and watching LOL doll YouTube™ videos. She has a TV in her bedroom and likes watching it whenever she is allowed. Grandma doesn't like YouTube. Gita's best friend in school is Abbie. Gita thinks Abbie is cool because she has brilliant shoes, makes her laugh, and is kind to her. Her favourite teacher is Ms. Smart because she helps her with maths. Gita hates maths but loves swimming lessons and hydrotherapy. Gita would like to be very rich and buy everyone ice cream and a necklace for her mum. After the call, Aesha was asked to fill in an I-ASC 'about me' form (https://iasc.mmu.ac.uk/wp-content/uploads/2019/04/I-ASC-About-me-blank.pdf) with Gita, and return the completed version in the post (Figure 2.3).

Jamie also made a phone call to Gita's main classroom teacher, Ms. Wilson, who described Gita as very sociable and great fun, with a clear yes/no response. Ms. Smart, the teaching assistant, indicated that Gita required an electronic communication aid, but Ms. Wilson had not used one before. Gita already

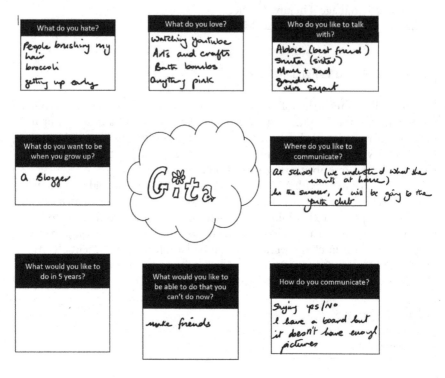

Figure 2.3 'ALL about Gita'

had a picture-symbol book but needed significant help to use it. Ms. Wilson did not like it and was concerned that Gita was somewhat lazy and preferred people to speak for her. Ms. Smart helped Gita to choose the picture symbols for her communication book. Gita's sister Smita had helped Gita put more picture symbols in it at home. Ms. Wilson understood that speech and language therapy would help Gita talk.

Step 2. Prioritise Information

The I-ASC Communication System Assessment Planning Checklist can be a helpful tool in synthesising available information to establish priorities for an assessment (see https://iasc.mmu.ac.uk/wpcontent/uploads/2021/11/i_asc_ communication_system_assessment_planning_checklist_oct_21.pdf). Gita's completed checklist can be found at https://iasc.mmu.ac.uk/wp-content/uploads/2021/ 11/I-ASC-Communication-System-Assessment-Planning-Checklist-Gita-example.pdf.

Before meeting Gita, information from the referral letter, phone calls, and the I-ASC 'About me' template provided an understanding of Gita, her family, and the context, information important to both assessment and intervention planning. Completing the assessment planning checklist brings together all the information and also highlights what gaps remain. In Gita's context, it was used to identify three priorities for the first stage of assessment. The following section outlines each of these priorities and the rationale for choosing them as the starting point for an AAC assessment.

Priority 1: A comprehensive understanding of Gita's receptive and expressive language abilities and her communication abilities across all modalities (e.g., speech, gesture, using symbols). All communication aid assessments should include detailed summaries of current language and communication skills. There was no existing language assessment for Gita, so this element is a critical first step to inform the AAC assessment.

While it can be challenging to assess children who use or may need to use AAC, a comprehensive review of language skills provides an essential foundation for other decisions. Observational evidence (including descriptive information from family and school) and informal assessment tasks can be used to probe different skills (e.g., Batorowicz et al., 2018; Deliberato et al., 2018; Murray et al., 2018; Smith et al., 2018; Stadskleiv et al., 2018; von Tetzchner et al., 2018). Some formal language assessment tools, such as the Test of Reception of Grammar (Bishop, 2003); British Picture Vocabulary Scales (BPVS, Dunn et al., 2009); and C-BiLLT (Geytenbeek, 2008) involve limited motor demands and may be completed as specified in the standardisation protocols. Even if standardised administration must be adapted to suit an individual, precluding the use of standard scores, such tests can still offer helpful information about receptive and expressive language abilities.

Typically, children who use AAC employ a range of communication modes in different contexts and with different partners. It is important to gain a comprehensive understanding of their existing skills/aided skills to inform planning for how a new aid might enhance their communication. This process may help:

- Identify how communication abilities are viewed in different locations and help ensure aid recommendations complement existing communication systems such as those within the family.
- Identify what communication opportunities exist for the child or young person to learn how to use their AAC system and support them to achieve agreed goals.
- Identify the aspects of multimodal communication that are used and how they are prioritised in different locations (e.g., unaided communication may be used more at home and aided communication more in school).

A comprehensive language and communication abilities profile is an essential component of the AAC assessment for all children and young people. If the information is not already available, it should be planned for *before* considering specific devices to trial. With extremely limited information on Gita's linguistic and communication ability, assessment for a device could not continue until a language and communication profile was created. The first step after information gathering should always be to establish if a language and communication profile is available and, if not, plan to obtain one.

Current Clinical Context: Gita's Language and Communication Skills

Gita attended four appointments at her local SLT service for a language and communication assessment – a considerably longer process than an assessment of a child who can speak.

Areas of strength and of need are summarised below, and a more detailed language and communication profile can be found at this link: https://iasc.mmu.ac.uk/wp-content/uploads/2021/11/Gita-language-and-communication-profile.pdf.

Receptive Language Strengths and Needs

Gita's understanding of vocabulary was an area of relative strength. She was able to follow two- and three-element utterances, understand negatives (e.g., not), action words (e.g., kicking), and colours (e.g., red, yellow, blue). Gita had difficulty processing more complex utterances (four-element level), understanding constructs like *not only X but also Y*, and plurals. Her understanding of prepositions (e.g., behind, beside, in front of) appeared inconsistent.

Expressive Language and Communication Strengths and Needs

Gita was a multimodal communicator who engaged well and persevered to get her message across. She used spoken word approximations, vocalisations, gesture, facial expression, and a communication book to communicate. A key strength was her ability to combine modes of communication. Gita was observed to use her communication book when prompted, and she demonstrated the ability to combine one- and two-symbol utterances. Gita demonstrated strengths in using noun and noun-verb structures. In terms of needs, Gita mostly used unaided modes (e.g., facial expression, vocalisation, and gesture) and often relied on familiar partners to interpret her messages. When communication breakdown occurred, Gita tended to look to Aesha for support and used few strategies to repair the communication herself. She was also observed to rely on a limited range of word classes when using her communication book (nouns and noun-verb combinations).

Priority 2: A comprehensive understanding of the current AAC system. The information gathered suggested that Gita had a communication book, but it was used in a limited way. Her teacher was concerned that she didn't use the book out of laziness, and her mother indicated that it didn't have sufficient vocabulary. Missing information included what Gita or her teaching assistant thought about the book, or why Gita's teacher and mother held the views they expressed.

Understanding each person's view on the communication book and how it is used is important in informing the assessment process. Developing a good understanding of what is currently happening and why it is not working well supports effective planning for any new system and can help identify adaptations that could be made to the current book to make it more useful. It can also help prevent repeating the same mistakes with a new system and ensure the new system incorporates strengths and preferences from the existing system.

An I-ASC spidergram activity was carried out to ascertain each person's view on Gita's current communication book and to spark discussion around priorities across the team for any new system (see https://iasc.mmu.ac.uk/wp-content/uploads/2019/05/I-ASC-How-to-use-the-spidergram-resource.pdf). Using the spidergram, each team member (including Gita) rated the features of the existing communication aid.

The spidergram exercise illustrates clearly the similarities and differences of opinion about Gita's current communication book. There were broad levels of satisfaction with the type of graphic representation system. Other than Gita, all involved seemed unhappy with the amount of vocabulary available. Views on vocabulary organisation, ease of customisation/editing, ease of mounting and portability, and the general appearance of the current aid varied greatly. These factors required further exploration to understand these differences better, ensuring all perspectives were heard, considered, and reviewed. Most team members raised physical access as a concern, suggesting some specialist input was required from an occupational therapist to review Gita's current and future manual abilities. Gita used the knuckle of her little finger to point, which worked well for her current aid.

Priority 3: Identifying available resources and supports for funding a system and implementing a new system. Implementing any AAC system requires support and input from those around the child. Sometimes, systems are recommended without a clear plan for supporting the child and identifying who will take on different responsibilities. The information gathered suggested Gita had some good supports around her that could be harnessed (e.g., her sister already added symbols to her book), but a new system would require additional supports. Gita's teacher had never supported a child using an electronic communication aid before, so if such a device were recommended, training would be needed. Some AAC systems require more support than others, and it is crucial to plan who will take on support roles

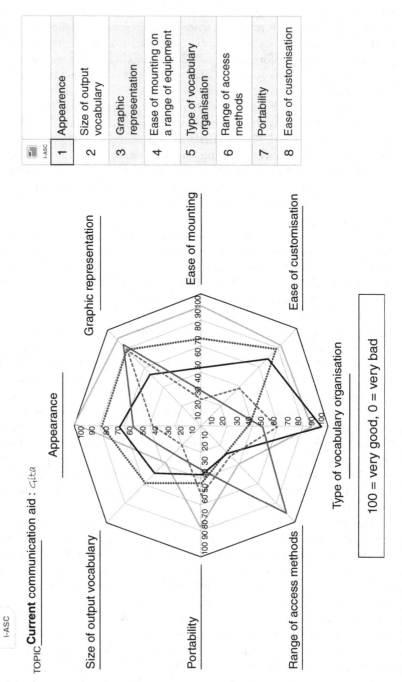

I-ASC	
1	Appearence
2	Size of output vocabulary
3	Graphic representation
4	Ease of mounting on a range of equipment
5	Type of vocabulary organisation
6	Range of access methods
7	Portability
8	Ease of customisation

Gita, Aesha, **Mrs Wilson,** Mrs Smart, **SLT**

TOPIC __Current__ communication aid : *Gita*

100 = very good, 0 = very bad

Figure 2.4 Prioritisation of communication aid attributes

when any aid is recommended. If support is a significant obstacle, training and intervention may need to be directed to addressing support before recommending an AAC system.

Choosing Roles and Responsibilities Checklist

The I-ASC Choosing Roles checklist (https://iasc.mmu.ac.uk/wp-content/uploads/2019/04/I-ASC-Choosing-roles-in-AAC-decision-making-and-implementation.pdf) helps identify the skills and abilities available across the team. Identifying roles that suit team members best will assist effective AAC support (Johnson et al., 1996). These roles are not profession- or family member–specific. They are open to any member of the team. Figure 2.5 illustrates what was agreed for Gita's AAC support team.

Choosing roles in AAC decision making and implementation: Gita's support network

Receiver of information: Aesha (Gita's mother) and Dr. Scott would like to receive a summary from the team about the outcomes of the assessment, with an overview of the short-, medium-, and long-term goals, including details of who has taken responsibility for delivery of the different aspects of the implementation plan.

Observer: Ms. Smart agrees she regularly spends time with Gita and can quietly observe and record/notice her communication behaviours as they occur.

Contributor: Ms. Wilson works with Gita and can offer information that would be useful to share, for example, academic skills, fine/gross motor skills, test results, and other classroom information.

Champion: Although not asked yet, Aesha wondered if Smita (Gita's sister) would be good in this role. Smita spends regular time with Gita and knows what is important to her in everyday life. She might like to share her experiences of how and what communication strategies may work well for Gita.

Coordinator: Ms. Smart agreed to seek out others' opinions about Gita's current and future communication needs, coordinating all the viewpoints. This coordinating role will ensure the decision-making team is well informed and can make the best decision with Gita.

Assessor: Jamie (the SLT) and Ms. Smart (an experienced teaching assistant) can carry out all or some aspects of the AAC assessment. Jamie (the SLT) will also approach occupational therapy regarding Gita's manual abilities.

Evaluator of (available) information: Jamie (the SLT) has agreed to lead on evaluating all the available information and data. However, Gita, Aesha, Smita, and Ms. Smart have agreed to help.

Active participant in implementation: Jamie (the SLT) is willing to lead the implementation process but will work closely with Ms. Smart and Smita. They are keen to work with Gita on her AAC skills and knowledge.

Figure 2.5 Summary of choosing roles debate

Step 3: Use the Information Collated to Guide Recommendations

At the end of the first stage of the assessment process, the relevant information on Gita enabled progression to the second stage of decision making. Here the focus was on what communication systems had the most appropriate features for Gita, synthesising the information to date, and evaluating the implications for Gita. It is generally appropriate to think about a system trial period to see what all those involved think about different system options. The I-ASC explanatory model (Judge et al., 2019; Lynch et al., 2019; Murray et al., 2019; Murray et al., 2020) can help highlight the range of elements considered for Gita and her team.

Child Characteristics

Gita was a strong multimodal communicator who used speech, gesture, and symbols to communicate. She primarily used single symbols to communicate and often needed prompting. Gita would benefit from an AAC system to support her expressive output and enable her to communicate more independently, particularly with less familiar partners. Gita also required a comprehensive literacy assessment and given her profile it was likely she would require specific supports to develop essential literacy skills (Dahlgren Sandberg et al., 2010; Smith, 2015; Smith et al., 2009).

Communication Aid Attributes

Gita knew the symbols on her communication book well, and it was important to retain this existing knowledge in a new system. A lot of fringe vocabulary had been added to her book in an ad hoc way. The core vocabulary available was limited. Her book required updating to systematise the vocabulary layout and expand the vocabulary. These recommendations should also be applied to any new system (Lund & Light, 2007; Schlosser & Lee, 2000; Stephenson, 2009; Trudeau et al., 2010). The look of the book and the new system were important to Gita, and she needed to be included in decisions related to these aesthetics.

Access Features

Gita used her communication book flat on her wheelchair tray and used her right little finger knuckle to point to the picture symbols. She seemed to have difficulty lifting her arm to knuckle point and sometimes knocked the book onto the floor, creating frustration. Further exploration was needed of where to optimally position the book and a new aid and how Gita should access them.

Ways of Working

A clear plan was developed of who would do what in the next stage. The discussion around roles and responsibilities helped bring Gita's teacher on board with supporting activities in class, an important consideration (Binger et al., 2012; Dietz et al., 2012). Gita's mother, Aesha, also understood how important it was for Gita to become more independent in communicating with those who did not know her well.

Transitions

The discussions highlighted the need to get a high-tech system in place and working well for Gita before she transitioned to secondary school. The assessment process also highlighted the need to support Gita in transitioning to more independent communication. The youth club was identified as a good place to focus on new communication opportunities (Bryen et al., 2010).

Available Resources

It was agreed that training on aided language modelling would be provided to Gita's family and school to scaffold how Gita might use her symbol-based supports. Her school indicated a willingness to fund an aid for Gita, but it would only be possible to use it at school. As agreed, Ms. Smart and Smita, along with Jamie, the SLT, developed a rota of activities to help everyone learn how to use the new aid and find old and new vocabulary. This timetable was designed to give Gita several short 'AAC lessons' each day.

Summary of Clinical Decisions

At the end of the first phase of the assessment, it was decided to immediately upgrade Gita's communication book and start modelling how to use the vocabulary. At the same time, a two-week device trial of a high-tech system was recommended. Upgrading the communication book offered Gita continuity with a familiar symbol system. On both the communication book and the trial device, symbols were reorganised syntactically, and additional vocabulary items were provided. The trial device offered Gita voice output to support independence and more options for access. A detailed plan was put in place to optimise the trial period and use the information gained to determine the next steps. A full review of physical access options with an occupational therapist was also planned.

Conclusion

This chapter outlines initial steps in an AAC assessment and detailed a range of resources that can be used to support those steps. Recent research suggests that some steps in AAC assessment may be omitted (Lynch et al., 2019;

Murray et al., 2019; Webb et al., 2019), and a review of competing considerations based on best assumptions may be used instead to drive decision making. While the initial recommendation from both a comprehensive assessment and a fast-tracked feature-matching process may be similar, a comprehensive assessment places the child and those closest to them in the driving seat of decision making. Taking time to explore person-specific issues and to consider resources and barriers leads to discussions where family and close staff members can take a central role in choosing and implementing the system (King et al., 2008). Through this collaborative way of working, it is possible to bring about change that will have lasting positive impacts for children who use AAC and their families (Goldbart & Marshall, 2004; Parette et al., 1999).

Acknowledgments

This research was funded by the National Institute for Health Research: Health Services & Delivery Research. Project reference number: 14/70/153. We would like to thank our co-researchers and collaborators (Prof. Juliet Goldbart, Simon Judge, Prof. Stephane Hess, Dr. David Meads, Stuart Meredith, Liz Moulam, Nicola Randall, Dr. Edward Webb, Helen Whittle), our participants, and advisors during the delivery and development of this research and associated outputs.

References

Batorowicz, B., Stadskleiv, K., Renner, G., Sandberg, A. D., & von Tetzchner, S. (2018). Assessment of aided language comprehension and use in children and adolescents with severe speech and motor impairments. *Augmentative and Alternative Communication*, *34*(1), 54–67. https://doi.org/10.1080/07434618.2017.1420689

Beukelman, D., & Mirenda, P. (Eds.). (2013). *Augmentative and alternative communication supporting children and adults with complex communication needs* (4th ed.). Paul H. Brookes.

Binger, C., Ball, L., Dietz, A., Kent-Walsh, J., Lasker, J., Lund, S., . . . Quach, W. (2012). Personnel roles in the AAC assessment process. *Augmentative and Alternative Communication*, *28*(4), 278–288. https://doi.org/10.3109/07434618.2012.716079

Bishop, D. (2003). *Test for reception of grammar-2*. Harcourt Assessment.

Bryen, D. Chung, Y., & Lever, S. (2010). What you might not find in a typical transition plan! Some important lessons from adults who rely on augmentative and alternative communication. *Perspectives on Augmentative and Alternative Communication*, *19*(June), 5–8.

Dahlgren Sandberg, A., Smith, M., & Larsson, M. (2010). An analysis of reading and spelling abilities of children using AAC: Understanding a continuum of competence. *Augmentative and Alternative Communication*, *26*(3), 191–202. https://doi.org/10.3109/07434618.2010.505607

Deliberato, D., Jennische, M., Oxley, J., Nunes, L. R. D. D. P., Walter, C. C. D. F., Massaro, M., . . . von Tetzchner, S. (2018). Vocabulary comprehension and strategies in name construction among children using aided communication. *Augmentative and Alternative Communication*, *34*(1), 16–29. https://doi.org/10.1080/07434618.2017.1420691

Dietz, A., Quach, W., Lund, S. K., & McKelvey, M. (2012). AAC assessment and clinical-decision making: The impact of experience. *Augmentative and Alternative Communication*, *28*(3), 148–159. https://doi.org/10.3109/07434618.2012.704521

Dunn, L. M., Dunn, D. M., Styles, B., & Sewell, J. (2009). *The British picture vocabulary scale III* (3rd ed.). GL Assessment.

Geytenbeek, J. (2008). *Computer-based instrument for low motor language testing*. www.c-billt.com

Goldbart, J., & Marshall, J. (2004). "Pushes and pulls" on the parents of children who use AAC. *Augmentative and Alternative Communication, 20*(4), 194–208. https://doi.org/10.1080/07434610400010960

Johnson, J. M. Baumgart, D., Helmstetter, E., & Curry, C. A. (1996). *Augmenting basic communication in natural contexts*. Paul H. Brookes Publishing Co. Inc.

Judge, S., Randall, N., Goldbart, J., Lynch, Y., Moulam, L., Meredith, S. . . . Murray, J. (2019). The language and communication attributes of graphic symbol communication aids – a systematic review and narrative synthesis. *Disability and Rehabilitation: Assistive Technology, 15*(6), 652–662. https://doi.org/10.1080/17483107.2019.1604828

King, G., Batorowicz, B., & Shepherd, T. A. (2008). Expertise in research-informed clinical decision making: Working effectively with families of children with little or no functional speech. *Evidence-Based Communication Assessment and Intervention, 2*(2), 106–116. https://doi.org/10.1080/17489530802296897

Lund, S. K., & Light, J. (2007). Long-term outcomes for individuals who use augmentative and alternative communication: Part II – communicative interaction. *Augmentative and Alternative Communication, 23*(1), 1–15. https://doi.org/10.1080/07434610600720442

Lynch, Y., Murray, J., Moulam, L., Meredith, S., Goldbart, J., Smith, M., . . . Judge, S. (2019). Decision-making in communication aid recommendations in the UK: Cultural and contextual influencers. *Augmentative and Alternative Communication, 35*(3), 180–192. https://doi.org/10.1080/07434618.2019.1599066

Murray, J., Lynch, Y., Goldbart, J., Moulam, L., Judge, S., Webb, E., . . . Hess, S. (2020). The decision-making process in recommending electronic communication aids for children and young people who are non-speaking: The I-ASC mixed-methods study. *Health Services and Delivery Research, 8*(45), 1–158. https://doi.org/10.3310/hsdr08450

Murray, J., Lynch, Y., Meredith, S., Moulam, L., Goldbart, J., Smith, M., . . . Judge, S. (2019). Professionals' decision-making in recommending communication aids in the UK: Competing considerations. *Augmentative and Alternative Communication, 35*(3), 167–179. https://doi.org/10.1080/07434618.2019.1597384

Murray, J., Sandberg, A. D., Smith, M. M., Deliberato, D., Stadskleiv, K., & von Tetzchner, S. (2018). Communicating the unknown: Descriptions of pictured scenes and events presented on video by children and adolescents using aided communication and their peers using natural speech. *Augmentative and Alternative Communication, 34*(1), 30–39. https://doi.org/10.1080/07434618.2017.1420690

Parette, P., VanBiervliet, A., & Hourcade, J. J. (1999). Family-centered decision making in assistive technology. *Journal of Special Education Technology, 15*(1), 45–55. https://doi.org/10.1177/016264340001500104

Schlosser, R., & Lee, D. (2000). Promoting generalization and maintenance in augmentative and alternative communication: A meta-analysis of 20 years of effectiveness research. *Augmentative and Alternative Communication, 16*(4), 208–226. https://doi.org/10.1080/07434610012331279074

Smith, M. M. (2015). Language development of individuals who require aided communication: Reflections on state of the science and future research directions. *Augmentative and Alternative Communication, 31*(3), 215–233. https://doi.org/10.3109/07434618.2015.1062553

Smith, M. M., Batorowicz, B., Sandberg, A. D., Murray, J., Stadskleiv, K., van Balkom, H., . . . von Tetzchner, S. (2018). Constructing narratives to describe video events using aided communication. *Augmentative and Alternative Communication, 34*(1), 40–53. https://doi.org/10.1080/07434618.2017.1422018

Smith, M., Sandberg, A. D., & Larsson, M. (2009). Reading and spelling in children with severe speech and physical impairments: A comparative study. *International Journal of Language & Communication Disorders, 44*(6), 864–882. https://doi.org/10.1080/13682820802389873

Stadskleiv, K., Batorowicz, B., Massaro, M., van Balkom, H., & von Tetzchner, S. (2018). Visual-spatial cognition in children using aided communication. *Augmentative and Alternative Communication, 34*(1), 68–78. https://doi.org/10.1080/07434618.2017.1422017

Stephenson, J. (2009). Iconicity in the development of picture skills: Typical development and implications for individuals with severe intellectual disabilities. *Augmentative and Alternative Communication, 25*(3), 187–201. https://doi.org/10.1080/07434610903031133

Trudeau, N., Sutton, A., Morford, J. P., Côté-Giroux, P., Pauzé, A. M., & Vallée, V. (2010). Strategies in construction and interpretation of graphic-symbol sequences by individuals who use AAC systems. *Augmentative and Alternative Communication, 26*(4), 299–312. https://doi.org/10.3109/07434618.2010.529619

van Niekerk, K., Dada, S., & Tönsing, K. (2017). Influences on selection of assistive technology for young children in South Africa: Perspectives from rehabilitation professionals. *Disability and Rehabilitation, 41*(8), 912–925. https://doi.org/10.1080/09638288.2017.1416500

von Tetzchner, S., Launonen, K., Batorowicz, B., Nunes, L. R. D. D. P., Walter, C. C. D. F., Oxley, J., . . . Deliberato, D. (2018). Communication aid provision and use among children and adolescents developing aided communication: An international survey. *Augmentative and Alternative Communication, 34*(1), 79–91. https://doi.org/10.1080/07434618.2017.1422019

Webb, E. J. D., Meads, D., Lynch, Y., Randall, N., Judge, S., Goldbart, J., . . . Murray, J. (2019). What's important in AAC decision making for children? Evidence from a best – worst scaling survey. *Augmentative and Alternative Communication, 35*(2), 80–94. https://doi.org/10.1080/07434618.2018.1561750

3 Supporting Emerging Communicators using AAC

Two Case Reports

Muireann McCleary and Yvonne Lynch

Introduction

Young children experiencing difficulty learning to speak and who communicate primarily using nonsymbolic means may be described as emerging communicators. Emerging communicators have not yet developed a reliable, symbolic way of expressing themselves (Dowden, 1999). Instead, they rely on nonsymbolic forms of communication, such as facial expression, pointing, body movement, and vocalisations (Garrett & Lasker, 2005). Their use of these forms means they are often dependent on others to interpret their meaning.

The presence of temporary or permanent difficulties with learning to speak can have wide-ranging implications for children's development and well-being (Romski et al., 2015). There are many reasons why children may have difficulty developing functional speech, including disabilities such as autism, cerebral palsy, and intellectual and developmental disabilities (Ryan et al., 2015). Despite the potential benefits of AAC supports for young children experiencing challenges in developing speech (Romski et al., 2015), many children under the age of three may not be offered these supports.

Sometimes those around the child may wish to wait and see how speech develops (Cress & Marvin, 2003), an approach that leaves children with limited ways of communicating at a critical stage of learning. There may be a belief that children need to demonstrate particular skills (e.g., object-picture matching) in order to benefit from AAC interventions (Cress & Marvin, 2003), although it is now well recognised that there are no prerequisite skills for learning to use AAC (Light & McNaughton, 2012). Finally, children may not receive AAC supports because of resistance among key stakeholders, including families, and a belief that implementing AAC implies giving up on speech (Oommen & McCarthy, 2015).

Parents and caregivers play a critical role in supporting communication and language development for all young children (Romski et al., 2005; Smith & Hustad, 2015). By working collaboratively with parents and caregivers, therapists can tailor AAC interventions to specific child and family needs (Parette et al., 2000). Many families already have effective ways of interpreting their child's communication. Collaborative discussion can ensure that any proposed

DOI: 10.4324/9781003106739-3

AAC supports draw on existing strengths within the family (Parette et al., 2000). Addressing the families' concerns about AAC in an open way can support the timely implementation of AAC for the best outcomes for children. Moving from a wait-and-see service delivery model to one where AAC supports are offered as soon as significant speech-language delays are identified provides young emerging communicators with the best chance of achieving their potential (Romski et al., 2015).

This chapter presents two case reports. These cases illustrate how children who initially present with similar skills may end up moving in very different directions. These cases also highlight the need to work collaboratively with families, recognise the family's strengths and needs, and deliver the intervention in a family-centred way. The timeline of intervention with both children is presented in Figure 3.1.

Case 1: Maria

Presenting Concerns

Maria was referred for a multidisciplinary team assessment by her paediatrician at 18 months with an evolving cerebral palsy. She attended for her first appointment with speech and language therapy, physiotherapy, and occupational therapy accompanied by her parents.

A case history was taken jointly by the team. Maria's parents outlined how shocked they were by her diagnosis, explaining that they had never imagined that they would attend a clinic with their two-year-old. Maria's hearing and vision had been assessed as being within normal limits. Her parents said that Maria could not sit unsupported and that she had "tight hands", two areas that were having an impact on her play opportunities. Maria's mother reported that feeding Maria was difficult and took a long time. Maria's parents said their goals for Maria were that she would walk, talk, and play with her toys.

Clinical Findings

Receptive Language Ability

The Receptive Expressive Emergent Language Scales 3 (REEL 3; Bzoch et al., 2003) is a parental checklist of receptive and expressive language skills. Maria's mother reported that Maria understood everything, that she responded to her name, understood "no", and looked to items on request. Some of the questions could not be answered as Maria's physical limitations meant she could not complete the activity described. Based on parental report Maria's receptive language skills scored in the very poor range. Maria's mother reported that Maria preferred highly coloured toys, which she tended to mouth. Maria was seated in her buggy for the session. She was not fully physically supported in this position and therefore assessment was limited by her loss of postural control.

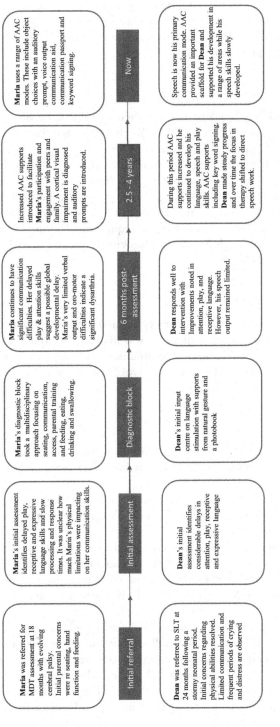

Initial referral

Maria was referred for MDT assessment at 18 months with evolving cerebral palsy. Initial parental concerns were re seating, hand function and feeding.

Dean was referred to SLT at 24 months following a stormy neonatal period. Initial concerns regarding physical abilities resolved. Limited communication and frequent periods of crying and distress are observed

Initial assessment

Maria's initial assessment identifies delayed play, receptive and expressive language skills and slow processing and response times. It was unclear how much Maria's physical limitations were impacting on her communication skills.

Dean's initial assessment identifies considerable delays in attention, play, receptive and expressive language

Diagnostic block

Maria's diagnostic block took a multidisciplinary approach focusing on seating, communication, access, parental training and feeding, eating, drinking and swallowing.

Dean's initial input centre on language stimulation with supports from natural gesture and a photobook

6 months post-assessment

Maria continues to have significant communication difficulties. Her delayed play & attention skills suggest a possible global developmental delay. Maria's very limited verbal output and oro-motor difficulties indicate a significant dysarthria.

Dean responds well to intervention with improvements noted in attention, play, and receptive language. However, his speech output remained limited.

2.5 – 4 years

Increased AAC supports introduced to facilitate **Maria**'s participation and engagement with peers and family. A cortical visual impairment is diagnosed and auditory prompts are introduced.

During this period AAC supports increased and he continued to develop his language, speech and play skills. AAC supports including key word signing. **Dean** made steady progress and over time the focus in therapy shifted to direct speech work.

Now

Maria uses a range of AAC modes. These include object choices with an auditory prompt, voice output communication aid, communication passport and keyword signing.

Speech is now his primary communication mode. AAC provided an important scaffold for **Dean** and supported his development in a range of areas while his speech skills slowly developed.

Figure 3.1 Timeline of interventions

She was observed to sustain attention in games initiated by the therapist. She appeared to respond to her name. Her response time to single-element verbal requests seemed slow. She was inconsistent in looking to a named object when two objects were presented.

Expressive Language Ability

Using the REEL 3, Maria's parents reported that she had a very limited range of open vocalic sounds ("ah" and "eh"). They reported that she was a happy girl who did not appear to get frustrated. She cried when tired, hungry, and sometimes after meals, placing her expressive language skills in the very poor range. Maria was largely silent during the session. She was interactive and appeared to enjoy people-focused games (e.g., peek-a-boo). She used open vocalisations ("aaah") and arching to request "more". Maria was observed to look to a person and then to an object to request objects. She appeared to have clear preferences for brightly coloured/moving items and to look to preferred items to indicate a choice.

Initial Clinical Hypothesis

Maria presented with delayed play, receptive and expressive language skills, and slow processing and response times. It was unclear how much Maria's physical limitations were affecting her communication skills, but it was clear that working as a team with Maria's parents would be key in clarifying the clinical picture.

First Steps

The multidisciplinary team met with Maria's parents to discuss the assessment outcome and to plan intervention. Key points of feedback included:

- Maria would benefit from adapted seating and exploration of different access methods (e.g., switch access or eye-gaze) to enhance her ability to participate in activities.
- Maria's language delays and communicative strengths were outlined. The benefits of introducing AAC to facilitate communication skill and language development and to promote communication were discussed.
- An assessment of Maria's feeding skills was recommended.

Maria's parents were very upset at the feedback saying that they had understood that Maria might have difficulties walking but had not realised that she might also have issues with hand function, feeding, and her speech. A team appointment was arranged for a week later to allow for further discussion and to develop an intervention programme. Following this initial appointment, the team shared the meeting outcomes with Maria's paediatrician and social worker.

Diagnostic Intervention

At the next meeting, the team worked with Maria's parents to identify the focus of an initial block of diagnostic intervention. Seven areas were targeted, each overlapping in impact.

1. ***Seating and positioning***: Without appropriately supportive seating, Maria was unable to engage in play activities. Three different positioning options were identified: a corner seat, a stander, and a wheelchair, providing Maria with positional support for a range of activities.

2. ***Analysing Maria's everyday communication experiences***: Communication logs are a useful clinical tool to gather detailed information about communication interactions, including information about opportunities to communicate, methods used, and the success of communication interactions (see Appendix 3.1). Maria's parents completed communication logs at home, which indicated that her needs were often anticipated. Many of her interactions appeared to be responsive and to signal pleasure or enjoyment (e.g., crying to signal tiredness or a desire for a change of activity). This information identified a need for training for Maria's parents to reduce their anticipation of her needs and create opportunities for Maria to develop her communication system, for example, through offering Maria choices.

3. ***Developing choice making and interaction opportunities:*** Maria's parents were asked to make a list of her likes and dislikes and to gather a bag of items that represented both. These items were for use in developing choice-making skills. Her parents were also asked to photograph Maria's important people and the objects from her choice bag. A photobook was developed with four photos on each page to help provide a reference point for conversation. This book allowed communication partners to engage with Maria on topics of interest to her (e.g., talking about people known to her), thereby increasing participation opportunities.

4. ***Access options:*** Due to her motor limitations, Maria was unable to physically manipulate objects or to engage in play. Working with Maria and her parents, the occupational therapist recommended she use a hand-switch to access toys. Using this switch Maria could activate toys, for example by pressing a switch to start a toy or to turn on music.

5. ***Developing interaction opportunities:*** Incorporating advice from Maria's occupational therapist, a single message voice output communication aid (VOCA) activated by hand-switch was recommended to facilitate Maria's participation in activities. A single message could be recorded at one time on this device allowing Maria to be an active participant in activities. Use of the device was modelled in therapy and a list of ideas for using the device was provided to Maria's parents.

6. ***Parent training:*** Recognising the key role communication partners have in AAC interventions, training for Maria's parents formed a part of all sessions. Her parents were supported to develop their skills in offering

choices, modelling choice making, waiting for and observing Maria's responses, and interpreting and labelling her responses.

7. **Team assessment of Maria's feeding, eating, drinking and swallowing (FEDS):** This assessment is not reported here as it does not directly relate to the focus of this chapter.

Because of Maria's multiple needs, an interdisciplinary approach to intervention was most appropriate. A plan was provided, combining therapy goals in a functional way that minimised the parental workload.

Progress

Over the next six months, Maria's mother joined the clinic's parent and toddler group and reported she found the support invaluable. She gained friendship and advice and learned from the experience of other parents. Following the parent training, both parents changed the way they interacted with Maria. They waited for Maria to signal a preference before responding to her and watched carefully to ensure they were interpreting her choices correctly. Maria made progress in choice making and could make nondirected choices of two objects (i.e., if offered two objects, Maria chose one). She was inconsistent in choices at a self-directed level; for example, if given a choice of a preferred item (teddy) and a nonpreferred item (truck) Maria did not consistently look to her preferred item. Use of an auditory prompt (i.e., labelling choices as they were presented) seemed to help and she expressed upset if given a nonpreferred item. Maria did not demonstrate interest in photographs. She enjoyed using the single-message VOCA to request continuation of games and she also enjoyed using her hand-switch to control cause-effect movement and brightly coloured toys. Her vocalisations remained limited to open vocalic sound making. Receptively, Maria remained inconsistent in her response to single-element requests such as *"where is the dolly?"* (with a choice of two objects).

Clinical Hypothesis After Maria's Initial Six-Month Intervention Period

Despite her progress in the six months of intervention, Maria continued to present with significant communication difficulties. Her delayed play and attention skills suggested a possible global developmental delay. Maria's very limited verbal output and oro-motor difficulties indicated a significant dysarthria.

Feedback to Maria's Parents

At a team review with Maria's parents, her continued significant delays in communication, as well as receptive and expressive language, were discussed. AAC was discussed with Maria's parents, both as a tool to help her to understand her environment and to provide her with a means to engage with her environment. The team recommended the use of objects to systematically and consistently represent items, people, or events to help Maria understand what might happen next (e.g., a sponge presented before bath time). The team also recommended offering Maria object choices to allow her to control and engage with her environment. Maria's parents were very upset and asked if the team was giving up on speech. They were reassured that the introduction of further AAC modes with Maria would not negatively affect her speech development. The importance of providing Maria with ways to communicate was highlighted and her parents were given reading material to take home. A further appointment to discuss their concerns was also offered.

Maria's preference for bright toys and movement-based activities in the diagnostic intervention block was raised by the team. Team members observed Maria benefitted from an auditory prompt to assist her choice making. These observations led the team to query whether Maria might have cortical visual impairment. Maria's parents had also noted her limited use of her vision, and so a referral for a functional visual assessment was made. Additionally, given Maria's complex presentation, it was agreed that a referral for a cognitive assessment would assist in identifying appropriate school placement for Maria.

Progress From 2.6–4 Years

On assessment of her functional vision, Maria was found to have cortical visual impairment (CVI). CVI is a visual impairment occurring in the visual processing centres of the brain (Roman-Lantzy, 2007). Cognitive assessment that traditionally relies on verbal, motor, and visual skills was challenging and time consuming, due to Maria's complex profile. Following the administration of parental reporting scales and observational scales, the psychologist diagnosed a global developmental delay.

Maria commenced at a special preschool for children with multiple disabilities. At the time of writing, Maria was using a single-message VOCA to engage in classroom activities, control activities, and bring news to and from home and school. She had a communication passport that detailed her communication systems and guidelines for communication partners. Objects of reference were introduced in a systematic way to assist Maria to process, understand, and engage in activities. A basic key word sign vocabulary was being used in the classroom and at home with Maria to support her receptive language development (see timeline summary in Figure 3.1). Key word signing refers to the provision of manual signs alongside spoken language to promote linguistic and communication skill development (Glacken et al., 2018). Despite Maria's parents' initial reservations about using AAC, they both attended key word sign training and found it a beneficial strategy at home.

At the time of writing, Maria had developed a consistent eyes-up response to indicate "yes" or a desire for continuance. Modelling of a head shake for "no" or "I don't like" was being undertaken by communication partners. Maria was offered choices of two objects at a nondirected/self-directed level throughout the day, with an auditory prompt using movement of the items to attract her visual attention. Communication partner training had been undertaken in the preschool. Progress was ongoing in all aspects of her communication and development.

Case 2: Dean

Presenting Concerns

Dean was referred to speech and language therapy at 24 months by his pae-diatrician, who reported that Dean had a stormy neonatal period. An early MRI scan indicated that Dean was likely to have a significant evolving physical disability. However, Dean made unexpected progress meeting his gross motor milestones and was fully ambulant. Of concern was Dean's behaviour, with frequent and extended periods of crying and distress reported.

Clinical Findings

Dean attended with his mother, Patricia, who reported that the period sur-rounding Dean's birth and early life had been traumatic, and she remained very concerned about Dean's future. She had limited support in caring for Dean, and was experiencing a lot of stress.

In the play-based observation, Dean was busy, picking up toys and objects and moving away again after a few seconds. He engaged with a play activity for up to a minute, followed his own interests, and tended to scream when redirected in play. Patricia reported that Dean's behaviour and communica-tion in the clinic were typical of how he behaved at home. These observa-tions suggested that his attention and listening skills were delayed for his age. At two years, it would be expected that he would be able to concentrate on a play activity of his choosing (Cooper et al., 1978). Furthermore, Dean's play interactions indicated he did not have the attention and listening skills to engage with a standardised assessment. The play observation was sup-plemented with a parental reporting scale to gain insight into his receptive and expressive language skills. The REEL Scale-3 (Bzoch et al., 2003) was completed with Patricia.

Receptive Language Ability

Dean attained a receptive ability score of 72 (poor range). Patricia reported that Dean showed understanding of family members' names, common words like "bye-bye", simple commands like "Let's go", and responded to music and singing with body movement (skills that typically emerge at 7–12 months of age). She reported that Dean did not respond to "no", could not listen for one minute while objects or pictures were named, and did not look in the direction of familiar objects when named (skills that typically emerge at 7–12 months of age).

Expressive Language Ability

Dean attained an expressive ability score of 65 (very poor range). He mostly communicated by crying and tantrums, by bringing Patricia to what he wanted, or pointing to objects. She reported he had some word approximations but that the meaning of these word approximations varied. In the appointment, Dean pointed and vocalised on 10 occasions, although his intended meaning was not always clear. He was observed to use /bi/ to label the ball, one of his favourite toys. However, some inconsistencies and vowel changes were observed with ball realised as /bi/, /dʌ/ and /bɔ/. Some groping behaviours were noted when producing sounds. The vocalisation "uh, uh" appeared to be used for several meanings and in combination with a pointing gesture. Patricia reported that she felt Dean was experiencing frustration and that his tantrums might be related to not being understood.

Oro-motor Skills and Observations

It was not possible to conduct an oro-motor assessment, but Dean was observed to have an open mouth posture and saliva loss to the level of his chest, with irritated skin on his chin.

Initial Clinical Hypothesis

Dean presented with considerable delays in the domains of attention, play, and receptive and expressive language. However, it was unclear why the delays occurred. Supports were needed immediately to help Dean and Patricia while the team continued to learn more about his skills and needs. A dynamic assessment approach was used to explore Dean's response to intervention. In dynamic assessment, the speech and language therapist (SLT) uses functional activities and provides different supports (such as scaffolding and modelling) and evaluates the child's response and skills to determine a child's potential to learn (Lund et al., 2017).

First Steps

Patricia was invited to the clinic without Dean. Dean's assessment results were shared, and it was explained that Dean's attention, play, receptive, and expressive language skills were all at an early stage of development. Patricia asked if Dean would ever learn to talk and then became visibly upset. The SLT acknowledged that the results were upsetting. She then answered Patricia's question in a truthful and straightforward manner. It was not known whether Dean would learn to talk, but he urgently needed communication supports, to alleviate the frustration he was likely experiencing.

Diagnostic Intervention

The intervention process initially focused on four key areas:

1. ***An early language stimulation programme focused on building joint attention***: As Dean was missing the early foundation skills for language learning, a parent-implemented programme of language stimulation was carried out using child-led play activities.
2. ***Analysing Dean's everyday communication and experiences with communication breakdown:*** Patricia was asked to keep a communication log for two days. The communication log provided insight into Dean's communication and informed intervention planning (e.g., the log helped identify opportunities for offering Dean choices and for modelling gestures to support understanding and expression). Patricia continued to update the communication log, noting challenges and progress. The log provided ongoing guidance in planning intervention (see sample log, Appendix 3.1).
3. ***Creating a photobook:*** A photobook of Dean's favourite objects, people, and places was created (see Figure 3.2). The photobook was used to engage Dean, build joint attention (talking about his favourite things), and facilitate communication (augmenting his vocalisations and gestures, repairing communication breakdown).
4. ***Exploring additional ways that Patricia could access support:*** A referral to social work was made with Patricia's consent. Following this referral, Patricia joined a parent and toddler group, gaining support from other parents.

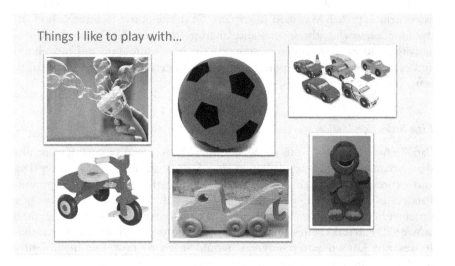

Figure 3.2 A photobook of Dean's favourite objects

Introducing AAC supports in a low-key way was important for this family. It allowed Dean to access the supports he needed in a way that was sensitive to Patricia's emotional state. The photobook was described simply as a photobook, and therapy initially focused on idiosyncratic gesture rather than a formal sign system.

Progress

Over the next 6 months, Dean made rapid progress in some areas and minimal progress in others. He quickly adopted the gestures, using them consistently to communicate. The photobook became one of his preferred shared activities with Patricia. Dean's attention skills improved, he engaged in joint play for a few minutes, and tolerated some adult intervention in play. He remained active but could sustain short bursts of attention in play. Some early symbolic play emerged. Patricia also reported that his behaviour had improved. Continued use of the log suggested that his behaviour was in part related to frustration with communication. As his communicative repertoire increased, the tantrums decreased. However, his speech remained severely limited. He used similar sounds for many meanings and had approximately three consistent word approximations. He also appeared to be self-conscious of his speech and was reticent to engage in sound play activities.

Clinical Hypothesis Following Dean's Initial Intervention Period

Despite the progress Dean made, his speech-language needs remained significant. It seemed increasingly unlikely that his difficulties were related to a significant learning or social communication disorder and more probable that there was a motor speech component to his speech profile, although it was not yet possible to assess him formally. Frustration related to his communication challenges also appeared to have affected Dean, limiting his progress. Once this frustration was addressed, rapid progress was observed in many areas, although his speech skills remained significantly affected. At this stage, it was decided that more formal AAC supports were needed.

Meeting with Patricia

Patricia was invited to discuss Dean's progress without Dean present. Dean's progress in attention, play, and understanding was highlighted. Dean's more limited means of expressing himself and his slow progress in developing speech was also discussed. It was explained that his speech skills were unlikely to meet his communication needs in the short to medium term. It was suggested that Dean would benefit from more formal AAC supports. As Dean had rapidly learned several idiosyncratic gestures, a key word signing programme was recommended (Glacken et al., 2018). Patricia appeared upset and asked if learning sign meant Dean was not going to talk. It was important to be honest with Patricia: although there were positive signs related to Dean's progress, it was unclear how his speech would develop. He needed more ways to express himself. The research evidence was also discussed and it was explained that AAC supports would not negatively impact his speech development (Cress & Marvin, 2003). Patricia agreed to attend a key word signing training programme.

Progress From 2.5–4 Years

Following the key word sign training, Dean and Patricia began using the signs at home. Dean's expressive sign vocabulary rapidly expanded. While key word signing was working well at home, Dean had recently started at créche as Patricia had returned to work outside the home. It was agreed that a créche visit would be carried out. The créche staff were very supportive of Dean, but had little experience of children like him and were unfamiliar with key word signing. Due to the number of staff involved and staff turnover, engineering the environment with picture supports was undertaken to enhance communication in that context. Dean continued to attend speech and language therapy with a continued focus on AAC, attention, listening, and receptive language skills. Over time, speech skill development became a greater focus. Dean's speech developed slowly but steadily. As he approached school-age, speech became his primary mode of communication, although he continued to require intensive speech work for an extended period (see Figure 3.1).

Conclusion

These two cases demonstrate how children who initially present as emerging communicators may follow different clinical pathways. For both, the early introduction of AAC served a vital function, reducing frustration for Dean and providing opportunities for participation and engagement for Maria. Introducing AAC early facilitates language and communication skill development (Cress & Marvin, 2003). Dynamic assessment allows evaluation of the emerging communicator's response to intervention (Lund et al., 2017). This response provides indicators of the potential role of AAC for the child (i.e., whether it will support expression while speech is developing, or if it will be the main form of expression). Central to the successful introduction of any AAC system is clear communication and close collaboration with communication partners. The role of these significant partners in fostering AAC systems (Calculator, 1997) and in facilitating maximum generalisation and reinforcement of communication skills is critical.

References

Bzoch, K. R., League, R., & Brown, V. L. (2003). *Receptive-expressive emergent language scale test* (3rd ed.). Pro-Ed.

Calculator, S. (1997). Fostering early language acquisition and AAC use: Exploring reciprocal influences between children and their environments. *Augmentative and Alternative Communication, 13*(3), 149–157. https://doi.org/10.1080/07434619712331277968

Cooper, J., Moodley, M., & Reynell, J. (1978). *Helping language development: A developmental programme for children with early learning handicaps.* Edward Arnold.

Cress, C. J., & Marvin, C. A. (2003). Common questions about AAC services in early intervention. *Augmentative and Alternative Communication, 19*(4), 254–272. https://doi.org/10.1080/07434610310001598242

Dowden, P. A. (1999). Different strokes for different folks. *Augmentative Communication News, 12,* 7–8.

Garrett, K., & Lasker, J. (2005). Adults with severe aphasia. In D. R. Beukelman & P. Mirenda (Eds.), *Augmentative and alternative communication: Supporting children and adults with complex communication needs* (3rd ed.). Brookes Publishing Co. http://aac.unl.edu/

Glacken, M., Healy, D., Gilrane, U., Gowan, S. H.-M., Dolan, S., Walsh-Gallagher, D., . . . Jennings, C. (2018). Key word signing: Parents' experiences of an unaided form of augmentative and alternative communication (Lámh). *Journal of Intellectual Disabilities, 23*(3), 327–343. https://doi.org/10.1177/1744629518790825

Light, J., & McNaughton, D. (2012). The changing face of augmentative and alternative communication: Past, present, and future challenges. *Augmentative and Alternative Communication, 28*(4), 197–204. https://doi.org/10.3109/07434618.2012.737024

Lund, S. K., Quach, W., Weissling, K., McKelvey, M., & Dietz, A. (2017). Assessment with children who need augmentative and alternative communication (AAC): Clinical decisions of AAC specialists. *Language, Speech, and Hearing Services in Schools, 48*(1), 56–68. https://doi.org/10.1044/2016_lshss-15-0086

Oommen, E. R., & McCarthy, J. W. (2015). Simultaneous natural speech and AAC interventions for children with childhood apraxia of speech: Lessons from a speech-language pathologist focus group. *Augmentative and Alternative Communication, 31*(1), 63–76. https://doi.org/10.3109/07434618.2014.1001520

Parette, H. P., Brotherson, M. J., & Huer, M. B. (2000). Giving families a voice in augmentative and alternative communication decision-making. *Education and Training in Mental Retardation and Developmental Disabilities, 35*(2), 177–190. www.jstor.org/stable/23879942

Roman-Lantzy, C. (2007). *Cortical visual impairment: An approach to assessment and intervention.* AFB Press, American Foundation for the Blind.

Romski, M., & Sevcik, R. A. (2005). Augmentative communication and early intervention. *Infants & Young Children, 18*(3), 174–185. https://doi.org/10.1097/00001163-200507000-00002

Romski, M., Sevcik, R. A., Barton-Hulsey, A., & Whitmore, A. S. (2015). Early intervention and AAC: What a difference 30 years makes. *Augmentative and Alternative Communication, 31*(3), 81–202. https://doi.org/10.3109/07434618.2015.1064163

Ryan, S. E., Shepherd, T., Renzoni, A. M., Anderson, C., Barber, M., Kingsnorth, S., . . . Ward, K. (2015). Towards advancing knowledge translation of AAC outcomes research for children and youth with complex communication needs. *Augmentative and Alternative Communication, 31*(2), 137–147. https://doi.org/10.3109/07434618.2015.1030038

Smith, A. L., & Hustad, K. C. (2015). AAC and early intervention for children with cerebral palsy: Parent perceptions and child risk factors. *Augmentative and Alternative, 31*(4), 336–350. https://doi.org/10.3109/07434618.2015.1084373

Appendix 3.1

Sample Communication Log

This log of Maria's communication will help us to identify how Maria is communicating her messages and where she is having difficulties.

Please complete this log at home so that we can get a full picture of Maria's daily communication.

Please add in as much detail as possible about Maria's communication.

All of this information will be used in developing communication systems for Maria.

Analysis of the communication log will help us identify:

1. What is working communicatively for Maria and how this may be built on.
2. Where there are opportunities for Maria to communicate and how these may be implemented.
3. Barriers to communication.
4. Training needs.

Date and time	Who communicated with	Where	Message	How Communicated	Success/not	If not successful – what happened
Example; 27-2-7am	Mammy	Kitchen – in her stander	Wanted her drink	Vocalised and looked to cup when mammy gave choice of cup or bowl	Yes – got her drink	No response
Example 27-2-8am	Mammy	Bedroom – lying on bed	Unclear	Crying – arching when clothes being put on	No	Stopped crying when dressed and downstairs

Analysis of Communication Log

In analysing the log, look at percentage of communication success across different themes, as shown below.

Time of Day	Communication Partners	No. of communication attempts	Percentage Success	Total percentage correct
Morning	Mammy	4	25	
	Daddy	2	50	33.3%
School time	Teacher	2	0	
	Assistant	4	100%	66.6%

4 Supporting Communication and Language Development in Preschool Children using AAC

Nancy Harrington, Carolyn Buchanan, Jennifer Kent-Walsh and Cathy Binger

Introduction

To become competent communicators, children who use aided AAC must be able to convey a range of novel messages for a variety of social purposes (Light & McNaughton, 2014). Novel messages are created through combining words and ideas into unique utterances. In preliterate children, these words and ideas typically are represented using graphic symbols (e.g., photographs and line drawings). Although a graphic symbol may represent an entire phrase, use of preprogrammed phrases may limit the scope of communication. For example, a symbol of a house may be programmed to communicate MY ADDRESS IS 123 SYCAMORE STREET – helpful if a child is answering a question about where they live, but with limited potential for communicating other messages about home. With a symbol for *HOME*, and the syntactic knowledge to combine symbols, a child can communicate that they want to *GO HOME*, that a friend *WENT HOME*, or ask when *MOM* will be *HOME*. These uniquely distinct utterances offer increased power and specificity of meaning and support greater independence in communication.

Young children can combine graphic symbols into multisymbol utterances using both low-tech and high-tech communication systems (Binger Kent-Walsh, King, & Mansfield, 2017; Binger, Kent-Walsh, King, Webb et al., 2017; Kent-Walsh, Binger, & Buchanan, 2015; Tonsing et al., 2014). Interventions targeting specific morphosyntactic structures have involved a variety of elicitation techniques that can be used in isolation or in combination with one another. Through these interventions, children have demonstrated the ability to acquire a range of targeted structures, including early semantic relations (e.g., Binger, Kent-Walsh, King, & Mansfield, 2017; (Binger, Kent-Walsh, King, Webb et al., 2017; Tonsing et al., 2014), and more sophisticated structures like inverted yes/no questions (Kent-Walsh, Binger, & Buchanan, 2015) and bound grammatical morphemes (Binger, Kent-Walsh, King, & Mansfield, 2017; Binger, Kent-Walsh, King, Webb et al., 2017; Binger et al., 2011).

DOI: 10.4324/9781003106739-4

Interventions to Target Multisymbol Utterances

Interventions targeting multisymbol utterances can exploit a range of elicitation techniques. For example, aided modelling (i.e., providing a model on the child's aided AAC system as well as a spoken model of the target utterance) can be used to expand spoken and aided output (Binger & Light, 2007). Aided input has been shown to positively affect aided expressive language when used as a single technique, and when employed in combination with other techniques (O'Neill et al., 2018). Using contrastive targets, or pairing an incorrect example with an accurate target, are techniques that can be easily incorporated into interventions using aided modelling (Binger, Maguire-Marshall, & Kent-Walsh, 2011). However, even with aided models and the use of contrastive targets, children may provide an incomplete response. In that case, a communication partner might provide a contingent aided response that adds missing information to model a more complete production (Binger, Maguire-Marshall, & Kent-Walsh, 2011). For example, an interventionist might model *DOG DRIVE CAR* (and speak the grammatically complete, "The dog is driving the car") in response to a child utterance of *DOG CAR*. Another common technique is use of an expectant delay or wait time, where a communication partner asks a question or makes a comment and then waits for the person using AAC to respond; this wait time may also be paired with an expectant gaze. The pause allows increased processing time, but also indicates to the person using AAC that the partner is finished speaking and is waiting for them to take a turn in the conversation (Kent-Walsh, Murza et al., 2015; O'Neill et al., 2018).

The Graphic Symbol Utterance and Sentence Development Framework

As clinicians employ these discrete intervention techniques, they may find themselves struggling to identify sequential targets to foster progressive growth in multisymbol message construction. The Graphic Symbol Utterance and Sentence Development Framework proposed by Binger, Kent-Walsh, Harrington et al. (2020) conceptualizes the linguistic development of children who use graphic symbols to communicate and illustrates a developmental progression from early symbol use (Phase 1) to the construction of "adultlike sentences" (Phase 4; see Figure 4.1). This framework includes an early focus on syntax in intervention from the time children begin combining symbols (Phase 2). It is grounded in Hadley's (2014) sentence-focused framework and aligns with Fey's (2008) argument that syntax should be considered from the outset of a child's AAC development. Although the Graphic Symbol Utterance and Sentence Development Framework can be broadly viewed as a progressive stepwise sequence of developmental phases, boundaries between phases are flexible, progression through phases may not be linear, and domains may progress at different rates. As word class and lexical diversity have been shown

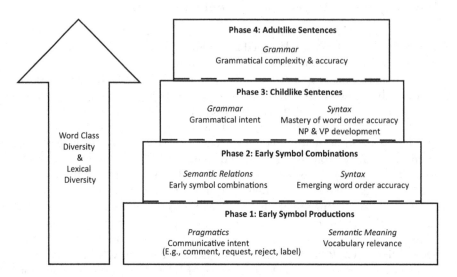

Figure 4.1 Graphic symbol utterance and sentence development framework (Reproduced from Binger et al., 2020) NP = noun phrase; VP = verb phrase

to expand throughout sentence development (Hadley et al., 2017), it is important to ensure that children who use graphic symbols have access to a range of vocabulary across word classes and across developmental phases to create a variety of novel utterances.

During Phase 1 of the model (Early Symbol Productions), children learn to use graphic symbols with both communicative intent (to request, comment, protest, etc.) and with semantic meaning as they develop single-word vocabulary. In Phase 2 (Early Symbol Combinations), they begin to combine symbols to express a variety of semantic relations with emerging word order accuracy. During Phase 3 (Childlike Sentences) the intended sentence is clear, there is mastery of word order accuracy, and the use of noun and verb phrases is evident. Phase 4 (Adultlike Sentences) sees the development of grammatical complexity and accuracy. The arrow on the left in Figure 4.1 highlights the ongoing development of word classes and lexical diversity as children's vocabulary grows.

Clinical Cases

In this chapter, "Jack" and "Carson" are pseudonyms used for two preliterate preschoolers who participated in clinical trials targeting aided sentence production using a graphic symbol AAC intervention approach. Jack participated in an intervention for preschoolers with severe speech impairments and typical receptive language skills, and Carson's intervention focused on young children with Down syndrome and significant speech impairments. Despite differences in presentation, these case reports illustrate how sentence development can be progressively targeted. They also highlight the overlap in intervention approaches as well as the diverse paths children can take along the Graphic Symbol Utterance and Sentence Development Framework.

Background and Presenting Concerns

Jack

Jack was four years and ten months old when he was referred to a university AAC clinic. Jack presented with intact receptive language skills and suspected childhood apraxia of speech (CAS). The Index of Augmented Speech Comprehensibility in Children, I-ASCC (Dowden, 1997) revealed 26% intelligibility for single words when contextual cues were provided and 6% intelligibility when only isolated words were presented.

Jack was a twin, born at 34 weeks' gestation. He spent his first three weeks in a neonatal intensive care unit (NICU). Jack was bottle fed, and no ongoing difficulties with feeding were reported. Developmental milestones for gross and fine motor skills were within normal limits, but language was delayed, resulting in referral to a speech-language pathologist at age two years and six months. Audiological assessment indicated hearing within normal limits. No structural abnormalities or dysarthria were evident during oral motor assessment. Jack had attended speech and language therapy on a biweekly basis since his initial referral, targeting expressive spoken language and speech production. As Jack became more verbal, it became evident that he was presenting with a severe speech production disorder. According to his parents, Jack was extremely frustrated when not understood, demonstrating anger, "giving up", and withdrawing from interactions.

Carson

Carson was five years and six months old when he was referred to participate in the clinical trial. Carson had a diagnosis of Down syndrome and had been attending speech and language therapy at his school for children with developmental disabilities since the age of two. Children with Down syndrome typically have reduced intelligibility compared with age peers, often negatively impacted by increased utterance length (Kent & Vorperian, 2013). They also often experience significant expressive communication delays, and early grammar and syntax have been identified as particular areas of significant and persistent difficulty (Romano et al., 2020).

Carson presented with normal birth and delivery, with no reported complications. Audiological assessment revealed hearing within normal limits and no vision difficulties were reported. He presented with hypotonia associated with Down syndrome, and delays in gross and fine motor development. Oral motor assessment revealed hypotonia, micrognathia, and difficulty with imitation of speech sounds for diadochokinesis and within isolated syllables and words.

When referred, Carson had been using sign language for approximately two years and presented with language and cognitive delays associated with Down syndrome. His sign vocabulary was limited to single signs, which he was reported to have dropped as he was becoming more verbal. Carson communicated in one- to three-word utterances with poor speech intelligibility (see Table 4.1). His parents and speech-language pathologist felt that aided AAC would be beneficial; Carson was due to begin kindergarten, and his family did not want communication difficulties to hinder his participation in school. He was reportedly becoming increasingly frustrated with his challenges in speech production; he had stopped speaking when not understood and would not speak at all in his preschool.

Diagnostic Assessment

All participants in the clinical trial were assessed for speech intelligibility, language skills, cognition, and motor skills (see Table 4.1). In addition, symbol assessment was completed to ensure that the participants could recognise and access the vocabulary on the graphic symbol displays. Finally, each participant completed a comprehension task to determine understanding of the basic semantic relation targets of the intervention: *agent-action-object, possessive-entity, attribute-object,* and *entity-locative.* Since the intervention focused on teaching the children to produce increasingly complex utterances for the targets, it was important to ensure that participants understood these basic semantic relations.

Clinical Findings

During baseline, Jack's production of graphic symbol utterances was assessed using Proloquo2Go with Symbol Stix© symbols on an iPad. A 42-location semantic-syntactic activity-specific grid display with modified Fitzgerald key colour coding (McDonald & Schultz, 1973) was employed. The display was arranged to facilitate sentence building with vocabulary organised by semantic categories from left to right. Likely subjects (e.g., pronouns, animal characters) were located on the far left of the display, followed by actions/verbs in the next column, prepositions/attributes in the next two columns, and likely objects/ nouns in the far-right column (Figure 4.2). Morphological endings -s and -ing were located at the bottom of the display and auxiliary verbs *am, is,* and *are* were adjacent to the verbs. Symbols that appeared on multiple displays (e.g., animal characters) appeared in the same location on each display.

Twenty-five video probes consisting of brief 10-second videos enacting sentences with potential for producing multiple targets were presented and Jack was asked to tell the examiner about the video. Examples of the targeted aided utterances included the following:

- *I AM WASHING PIG-S BOX:* agent-action-possessor-object
- *HAPPY ELEPHANT IS PUSH-ING THE YELLOW BED:* attribute-agent-action-attribute-object
- *LION-S DIRTY AIRPLANE:* possessor-attribute-entity
- *BIG DOG IS UNDER THE BLUE BOX:* attribute-entity-attribute-locative

Table 4.1 Participant Assessment Information

	Chronological Age	I-ASCC No Context/ Semantic Context	TACL-4 Receptive Language Index	CDI: Total No. of Words	Vineland Adaptive Behavior Scales – Third Edition	Leiter-3: Nonverbal IQ/ Composite Score	PPVT-5: Standard Score
Jack	4 yr. 11 mo.	6%/26%	128 (97th percentile)	Words and sentences: 670	Communication: 92 Social: 90 Motor: 93	115 (84th percentile)	N/A
Carson	5 yr. 8 mo.	19%/13%	59 (<1 percentile)	Words and gestures: 260	Communication: 56 Social: 72 Motor: 70	N/A	60 (.4 percentile)

Note. I-ASCC = Index of Augmented Speech Comprehensibility in Children (Dowden, 1997); TACL-4 = Test for Auditory Comprehension of Language – Fourth Edition (Carrow-Woolfolk, 2014); CDI = Communication Development Inventory (Fenson et al., 2006); Leiter-3 = Leiter International Performance Scale – Third Edition; PPVT-5 = Peabody Picture Vocabulary Test – Fifth Edition (Dunn, 2018).

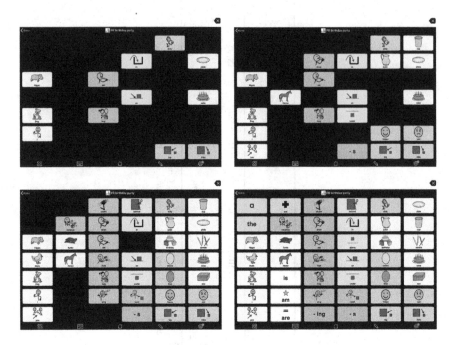

Figure 4.2 Sample displays for Birthday Party play routine (Proloquo2Go© with Symbol Stix©)

Jack was not expected to produce these types of utterances immediately, but rather to progress toward more complex utterances across the intervention. Progression might be from producing a one- or two-symbol utterance in baseline (*PIG BOX*), then expanding to include a grammatical marker (PIG-S BOX), then adding components such as agents and actions (*I WASH PIG-S BOX*), and eventually producing grammatically complete utterances (*I AM WASH-ING PIG-S BOX*).

Carson's baseline assessment was completed using a mediated play routine instead of video probes, as this was more developmentally appropriate for him. The same type of activity-specific displays for individual play routines were used (e.g., one display for playing with vehicles and another for baking), but with a reduced number of symbols. Given his cognitive and linguistic skills, Carson would have been overwhelmed by 42 symbols on a display; therefore, he started with a limited number of symbols visible, and the number of symbols was increased as his competency increased. All symbols remained in the same place as additional symbols were revealed, so that Carson would not have to "relearn" the location of symbols as he progressed (Figure 4.2). The initial "Step 1" display for Carson had 12 symbols to support grammatical multisymbol utterances: two agents/animals, the pronoun "I", two verbs, two prepositions (in, on), three adjectives (dirty, big, little) and two objects/toys. Carson's display was also arranged to facilitate sentence building with vocabulary organised from left to right.

Initially, Jack's aided expressive language was categorised in Phase 2 of the Graphic Symbol Utterance and Sentence Development Framework (Binger et al., 2020). He was able to independently produce multiword utterances, but he struggled with syntax and grammar. Typical baseline aided utterances included: *PUSH, BATHTUB MONKEY CAR, I -S SHAKE, LION-S DIRTY-S CAR.* Carson's aided expressive language was categorized in Phase 1 as he was producing one- to two-symbol aided utterances, such as *CAKE, CAKE PLATE, HIPPO CAKE.*

Diagnostic Intervention Using AAC Generative Language Intervention

The clinical trial intervention – "AAC Generative Language Intervention" (AAC-GLI) – was employed with Jack and Carson. The AAC-GLI comprises three components: (1) instructional techniques, (2) technology, and (3) context (Figure 4.3).

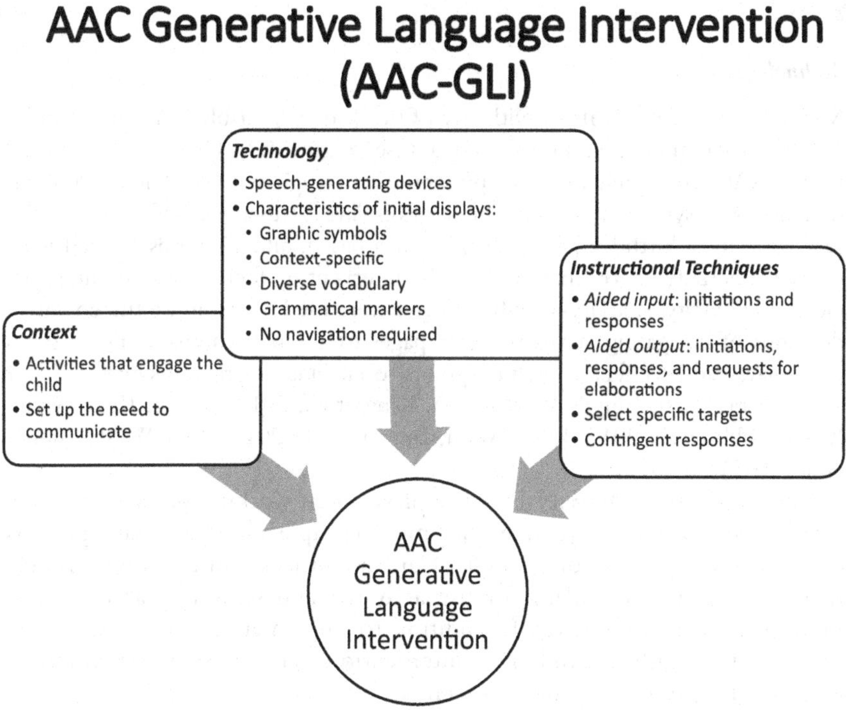

Figure 4.3 Components of AAC Generative Language Intervention

Instructional Techniques

AAC-GLI instructional techniques include aided AAC modeling/input, aided AAC use/output, selection of specific targets, and use of contingent responses. During aided AAC input or aided modeling, the adult models the targets, using grammatically complete spoken language plus an aided model of the target; the structure of the aided model is at or just above the child's current level of aided message productions and therefore may not be grammatically complete. Aided output involves prompting the child to produce targets (Romski et al., 2010). Aided modeling and aided output have proven effective in many AAC intervention studies to support language development (Binger et al., 2011, 2019; Binger, Kent-Walsh, King et al., 2017; Binger, Kent-Walsh, King, Webb et al., 2017; Binger & Light, 2007; Kent-Walsh, Binger et al., 2015; Romski et al., 2010). The selection of specific targets and use of contingent responses have been found to support both aided and spoken language semantic and pragmatic outcomes for children with autism and intellectual disabilities (Almirall et al., 2016), as well as sentence development (Binger et al., 2011, 2019; Binger, Kent-Walsh, King et al., 2017; Binger, Kent-Walsh, King, Webb et al., 2017; Kent-Walsh, Binger et al., 2015; Kent-Walsh, Murza et al., 2015).

Technology

Mobile devices such as iPads with any of the widely available AAC apps can be used to program context-specific displays (see Figure 4.2). On the displays used for the AAC-GLI, each word is represented by a single symbol. The child builds sentences one symbol at a time. Different displays are used for different activities (e.g., one for a birthday party, another for a farm), and all words needed for a particular activity are on that display. The intervention focused on building syntactic complexity. Activity-specific displays were used to minimise the cognitive demands of navigating across multiple pages to access vocabulary. These types of displays can be effective starting points to facilitate expressive syntax (Binger et al., 2011, 2019; Binger, Kent-Walsh, King et al., 2017; Binger, Kent-Walsh, King, Webb et al., 2017; Kent-Walsh, Binger et al., 2015; Kent-Walsh, Binger et al., 2015).

Children can use activity-based displays when working on syntax, while simultaneously learning to navigate more complex software with preprogrammed vocabulary. For example, Carson and Jack had iPads with robust core and fringe vocabulary for use at home and school, enabling communication across contexts. In addition to implementing these technologies directly with the children in intervention, technology instruction was provided for family members to facilitate the use of aided AAC systems at home, with an emphasis on both spoken and aided AAC models. This dual approach supported the children in using large core and fringe vocabularies to support semantic growth, while also minimising cognitive and operational demands to work on early phrase, clause, and sentence development – thereby supporting syntactic and grammatical growth. Regardless of communication mode, children need opportunities to develop semantic and grammatical skills simultaneously through the implementation of appropriate technologies.

Context

Since intervention contexts must be engaging and create a need to communicate, nine different motivating play routines were provided as options (shopping, birthday party, hide and seek, bed and bath, vet, desserts, lunch, farm, and vehicles). AAC-GLI elicitation techniques of employing contingent responses, open-ended questions, providing expectant delays, feigning ignorance, and offering binary choices were used to provide opportunities to communicate and to indicate the need to communicate. Table 4.2 includes detailed examples and video links to illustrate these elicitation techniques. Play-based AAC-GLI was provided for both boys twice weekly for 30-minute individual sessions at the university-based communication disorders clinic.

After every seven intervention sessions, a monthly measurement session occurred. Although each of the chosen play routines included unique vocabulary (e.g., *BUY* and *FOOD* for the shopping routine, vs. *EAT* and *CUPCAKES* for the dessert routine), some standard vocabulary was included on each display to assist learning: each display contained the same animals, the pronouns *I* and *YOU*, and at least two common adjectives, verbs, and nouns. All symbols on the display were reviewed at the start of each session. Puppets, small plastic animals, and other toys were modified to provide context for the targeted adjectives; for example, play materials included monkeys that were big, little, happy, sad, dirty, red, yellow, green, and blue.

Participant displays used at the outset of intervention were similar to those used in the baseline phase: Jack used the full 42-location display (see Figure 4.2) and Carson used a 12-location display (see Figure 4.2). For Carson to move up from Step 1 to Step 2 (21-symbol), he had to demonstrate semantic diversity in his symbol selection by independently using vocabulary across at least four out of five different word classes in two out of three sessions (Figure 4.4). These criteria were designed to ensure that Carson was learning the building blocks of sentence development. If he only learned to use a range of nouns, his multisymbol utterance productions would be limited, as most multiword utterances consist of more than one word class.

Table 4.2 AAC Generative Language Intervention Elicitation Techniques (With Video Links)

Technique	Rationale	Description or Example
Aided AAC modelling	Direct modelling of morphosyntactic structures aids learning of targets.	Clinician: "Look! Blue hippo is in the airplane" BLUE HIPPO IN AIRPLANE. Always accompany aided utterances with grammatically correct spoken language.
Repeat underlying structures across multiple targets	Helps child to focus on a particular linguistic structure.	Note: May do MANY of these – 10 or more – in a row when (a) teaching new structures, or (b) resolving word order issues. · HIPPO EAT CUPCAKE · DUCK EAT CUPCAKE · TURTLE EAT CUPCAKE · DOG EAT COOKIE · HIPPO EAT COOKIE
Open-ended questions	Encourages the child to make choices and describe the action of the play routine via the activity-based display.	"What would you like to bake today?" "Who do you want to play with today?"
Binary choice	Use when the child struggles to make choices based on open-ended questions; use also to highlight word order issues.	"Should red Hippo or red Duck help us with our baking?" "Does Dog want to ride in the blue train or the blue bus?"
	Use also to highlight word order issues	"Did you mean that you want Hippo red or red Hippo?"
Point to the toys	Draw the child's attention to things they can comment on; this may or may not be accompanied by spoken comments	Point to the truck to indicate that the child might want to get that out next.
Wait time	This gives the child the opportunity to initiate as well as respond. It also provides crucial processing time. For some children, you can look expectantly at the child so he knows you are excited to hear what he has to say.	Hold up the dirty truck and the red truck, look at the child, and wait for at least 5 seconds.
Feign ignorance	If the child is grabbing toys and/or gesturing instead of communicating via aided utterances, have the agents pretend to not understand, and direct the participant's attention back to the display.	Dog says: "I know you want me to do something, but I'm not sure what. Will you tell me with the iPad?"

Technique	Description	Example
Describe the action	Provide descriptions of the actions to provide the child with possible vocabulary, prompt aided utterances, and keep the routine going.	"I see Hippo hiding."
Spoken contrasts	This is a good technique to use when the child is making word order errors. We are directly highlighting that the child's job is to match her aided language with her spoken language (input-output asymmetry).	"Do you want to say, Horse in house or Horse house in? Oh, Horse in house, let's fix it."
Point to the symbols	This can help the child make longer, more complex utterances that are too challenging for her to create independently.	"Let's do it together. Hippo is big. Hippo (point to Hippo) is (point to is) big (point to big)." "I'm not sure who you're talking about. Tell me here." (Point to the display.)
Respond to all communicative attempts	Emphasize aided communication, but do not ignore the child's other communicative attempts. Respond and draw his or her attention back to the device.	Participant: DOG HIDE
Contingent responses	Use recasts, expansions, and extensions to respond to the child's communication attempts.	Clinician: "Yes, I see Dog is hiding." DOG IS HIDE -ING. Participant: HORSE Clinician: "That's happy Horse." HAPPY HORSE Participant: DUCK BARN Clinician: "Yes, that's Duck's barn." DUCK'S BARN
Use the message bar	Encourage the child to select the message bar at the top of the screen once his utterance is completed, so that he can hear his utterance and self-monitor accurate/inaccurate selections.	Say, "Tell me the whole thing" while pointing to the message bar.
Repair utterances	Allows opportunities to fix mistakes, often using binary choice	"Oh listen! Did you want to say, Horse in house or Horse house in? Oh, Horse in house, let's fix it." Assist the child with deleting the incorrect words as needed.

To step up participant must use 4 different word classes over 2/3 sessions with step-up criteria.

$$\text{Step 1} \longrightarrow 2 = 1 \text{ of each word class}$$

$$\text{Step 2} \longrightarrow 3 = 2 \text{ of each word class}$$

$$\text{Step 3} \longrightarrow 4 = 3 \text{ of each word class}$$

Figure 4.4 Step-up criteria

The intervention required a minimum dosage of modeling of target aided linguistic structures. All target basic semantic–syntactic structures (*agent-action-object, possessive-entity, attribute-object,* and *entity-locative*) needed to be produced at least twice by either the child or clinician within each 30-minute session. First-, second-, and third-person sentence types were also produced at least twice. Aided productions by the participant, the examiner, and co-constructed counted towards a minimum of 10 aided utterances per 30-minute play-based intervention session. All the clinicians' aided utterances were accompanied by grammatically correct spoken sentences. Clinicians generally provided aided models that were slightly longer than the boys' aided utterances to encourage utterance expansion. If the child made a word order error, the clinician corrected the word order instead of expanding the utterance. Contingent recasts, expansions, and extensions were used to respond to the participant's communication attempts (Binger & Light, 2007). For example:

PARTICIPANT: *DOG HIDE*
EXAMINER: "Yes, I see Dog is hiding." *DOG IS HIDE -ING.*
PARTICIPANT: *HORSE*
EXAMINER: "That's happy Horse." *HAPPY HORSE*
PARTICIPANT: *DUCK BARN*
EXAMINER: "Yes, that's Duck's barn." *DUCK-S BARN*

Procedural Fidelity

Procedural fidelity (Schlosser, 2002) for the delivery of the intervention was monitored using fidelity checklists. A random sample of 20% of the sessions was checked by trained coders. Procedural fidelity was calculated by taking the number of steps followed correctly, divided by the total number of steps multiplied by 100. Fidelity measures were 95% accurate for Jack and 97% accurate for Carson, indicating that the procedures were implemented consistently.

Progress

Both participants exhibited difficulty with word order accuracy in at least some utterances, so tracking the percent of unique multisymbol utterances that were produced with accurate word order provided one measure of development. Another measure was a modified version of mean length of utterance (MLU; Rice et al., 2010). Using MLU to track the development of graphic symbol utterances (i.e., MLUSym) is complicated (Binger et al., 2020). Two unique phenomena associated with aided language use are (a) relatively high rates of word order errors, and (b) selection of words irrelevant to the context (e.g., Binger, Richter et al., 2019). To address these issues, we used a modified MLUSym measure that only included utterances containing both relevant symbols and accurate word order. Specifically, a modified version of the mean of the three longest utterances (MLU3; Fenson et al., 2006), which is viewed as a measure of the upper bounds of a child's current expressive language abilities, was employed. This MLU3 in symbols, or MLUSym3, is hypothesized to provide a reasonable indication as to where the child's expressive language skills are headed.

Progress and Outcomes: Jack

Jack participated in the intervention program twice weekly over three months; the intervention was cut short due to the COVID-19 pandemic. At baseline, Jack was at Phase 2 of the Graphic Symbol Utterance and Sentence Development Framework (Binger et al., 2020) – producing multiword utterances but struggling with syntax. Clear, discernable word order was apparent for only 5% of his utterances; Jack appeared to be listing items and concepts he viewed in the video probes. His percentage of unique multisymbol utterances with discernable, accurate word order progressed from 5% to 76% after only one month of intervention (i.e., seven 30-minute play sessions) and had reached a level of 96% after three months of intervention (see Figure 4.5).

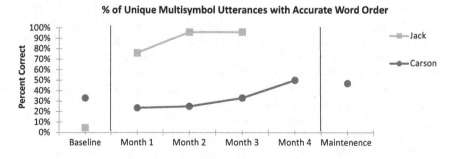

Figure 4.5 Results for production of unique multisymbol utterances with accurate word order

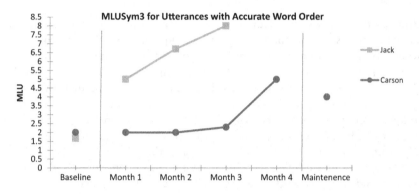

Figure 4.6 Results for MLUSym3 for utterances with accurate word order

At baseline, Jack's MLUSym3 was 1.67 (Figure 4.6); his three longest unique utterances without word order errors included two single-symbol utterances plus one accurate three-symbol utterance (1 + 1 + 3 = 5 symbols total; 5 symbols/3 utterances = 1.67). Jack's strong language comprehension skills likely supported his rapid progress to longer and more complex sentences. Some of his early productions included utterances such as *BATHTUB MONKEY COW* or *I -S SHAKE*. After only three months of intervention (i.e., approximately 10.5 hours), his MLUSym3 had grown to 8.0 (Figure 4.7). At this stage, Jack produced utterances that included the following: *I AM DRIVE -ING A TRAIN ON TRACKS, LITTLE DOG-S BIG GREEN AIRPLANE IS WIN -ING THE RACE,* and *DIRTY ICE-CREAM IN BIG TURTLE-S OVEN.*

Progress and Outcomes: Carson

Carson participated in the intervention program twice weekly over four months. Initially, Carson was at Phase 1. His percentage of unique multisymbol utterances with no discernable word order errors was 33%. (Figure 4.5). Carson used primarily nouns, so the initial focus was on word class diversification within *agent-action-object, attribute object, entity-locative,* and *entity-possessive* utterances. As Carson began to use more word classes, he progressed through the various "step-up criteria" outlined in Figure 4.4. During the fourth month of intervention, Carson was using displays with 42 symbols. As he progressed, he continued to demonstrate word order issues in his multisymbol utterances, but by month four, half his multisymbol utterances had accurate word order. Further, his MLUSym3 had increased from 2.0 to 5.0, and he was approaching Phase 3 in the Graphic Symbol Utterance and Sentence Development Framework, producing utterances including the following: *I SCOOP ICE-CREAM CONE, DUCK EAT BIRTHDAY CAKE,* and *I CHECK SICK*

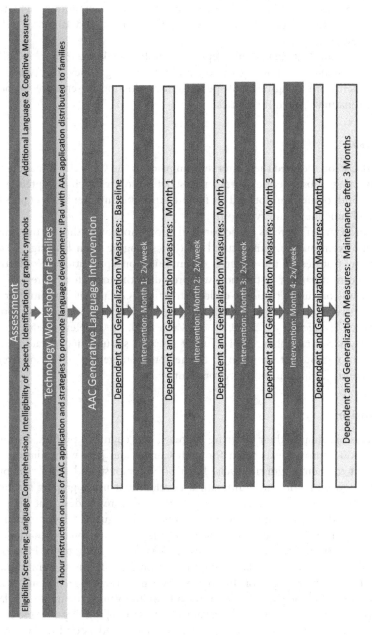

Figure 4.7 Timeline of Word-by-Word AAC Generative Language Intervention

TURTLE MOUTH. When Carson returned for a three-month maintenance check (i.e., no intervention for three months), his word order was still accurate approximately 50% of the time, but his MLUSym3 had dropped down to 4.0 (Figure 4.6). This highlights the need for consistent intervention, which is likely particularly important for children with cognitive and language delays such as Carson.

Both Jack and Carson's parents reported comfort with using the AAC iPad application at home following the technology training. They also perceived improvements in intelligibility of speech and production of sentences in both aided and natural speech modalities.

Limitations

Jack and Carson received their intervention prior to the COVID-19 pandemic. Unfortunately, subsequent closures and restrictions on research disrupted Jack's fourth month of intervention and his maintenance measurement (see Figure 4.7 for overall timeline of intervention).

Jack and Carson's parents participated in a four-hour workshop at the outset of the intervention program focused on topics ranging from language development to features of the selected communication application. No further communication partner instruction was provided; the focus for the rest of the program was on direct clinician-child instruction. Given that communication partner instruction has previously been linked to enhanced language outcomes for children (Binger et al., 2008; Kent-Walsh et al., 2009; Kent-Walsh et al., 2015; Hayes & Traughber, 2021), future research should incorporate parent training throughout intervention to further promote generalization of targets across natural communication environments.

Conclusions

In conclusion, despite their differing language and cognitive profiles, a similar intervention approach was taken for both Carson and Jack with adjustments as relevant to their linguistic levels. Both boys demonstrated significant progress in their semantic and grammatical development using graphic symbols. Predictably, Carson's improvement trajectory was more modest, but his progress demonstrates that children with cognitive and language delays can benefit from consistent AAC-GLI intervention. Both Jack and Carson are multimodal communicators and may not end up using AAC in the long term. However, during the preschool years, aided communication can facilitate communication and support participation in contexts where natural speech alone is not effective, bridging the gap between poor intelligibility and true expressive language potential. In addition to the severe speech unintelligibility of these boys, behaviors such as withdrawal and fear of not being understood can interfere with opportunity for socialization and academic participation and can result in adverse long-term effects. These adverse effects could be mitigated through approaches such as AAC-GLI, resulting in higher levels of linguistic competence leading to effective communication.

This work was supported in part by a grant from the National Institutes of Health (National Institute on Deafness and Other Communication Disorders). *Word by Word: Building Sentences with Preschoolers Who Use AAC.* Award No. *R01DC016321* (PI: C. Binger & MPI: J. Kent-Walsh).

References

Almirall, D., Distefano, C., Chang, Ya-Chih, Shire, S., Kaiser, A., Lu, X., . . . Kasari, C. (2016). Longitudinal effects of adaptive interventions with a speech-generating device in minimally verbal children with ASD. *Journal of Clinical Child & Adolescent Psychology, 45*(4), 1–15. https://doi.org/10.1080/15374416.2016.1138407

Binger, C., Kent-Walsh, J., Berens, J., Del Campo, S., & Rivera, D. (2008). Teaching Latino parents to support the multi-symbol message productions of their children who require AAC. *Augmentative and Alternative Communication, 24*(4), 323–338. doi:10.1080/07434610802130978

Binger, C., Kent-Walsh, J., Harrington, N., & Hollerbach, Q. C. (2020). Tracking early sentence-building progress in graphic symbol communication. *Language, Speech, and Hearing Services in Schools, 51*(2), 317–328. https://doi.org/10.1044/2019_LSHSS-19-00065

Binger, C., Kent-Walsh, J., King, M., & Mansfield, L. (2017). Early sentence productions of 3- and 4-year-old children who use augmentative and alternative communication. *Journal of Speech, Language, and Hearing Research, 60*(7), 1930–1945. https://doi.org/10.1044/2017_JSLHR-L-15-0408

Binger, C., Kent-Walsh, J., King, M., Webb, E., & Buenviaje, E. (2017). Early sentence productions of 5-year-old children who use augmentative and alternative communication. *Communication Disorders Quarterly, 38*(3), 131–142. https://doi.org/10.1177/1525740116655804

Binger, C., & Light, J. (2007). The effect of aided AAC modeling on the expression of multi-symbol messages by preschoolers who use AAC. *AAC: Augmentative and Alternative Communication, 23*(1), 30–43. https://doi.org/10.1080/07434610600807470

Binger, C., Maguire-Marshall, M., & Kent-Walsh, J. (2011). Using aided AAC models, recasts, and contrastive targets to teach grammatical morphemes to children who use AAC. *Journal of Speech, Language, and Hearing Research, 54*(1), 160–176. https://doi.org/10.1044/1092-4388(2010/09-0163)

Binger, C., Richter, K., Taylor, A., Williams, E. K., & Willman, A. (2019). Error patterns and revisions in the graphic symbol utterances of 3- and 4-year-old children who need augmentative and alternative communication. *AAC: Augmentative and Alternative Communication, 35*(2), 95–108. https://doi.org/10.1080/07434618.2019.1576224

Boisvert, M., Lan, R., Andrianopoulos, M., & Boscardin, M. (2010). Telepractice in the assessment and treatment of individuals with autism spectrum disorders: A systematic review. *Developmental Neurorehabilitation, 13*(6), 423–432. https://doi.org/10.3109/17518423.2010.499889.

Carrow-Woolfolk, E. (2014). *Test for auditory comprehension of language-Fourth edition (TACL-4)*. Pro-Ed.

Dowden, P. A. (1997). Augmentative and alternative communication decision making for children with severely unintelligible speech. *AAC: Augmentative and Alternative Communication, 13*(1), 48–59. https://doi.org/10.1080/07434619712331277838

Dunn, D. (2018). *Peabody picture vocabulary test, fifth edition (PPVT-5)*. Pearson Assessments.

Fenson, L., Marchman, V. A., Thal, D. J., Dale, P. S., Reznick, S. J., & Bates, E. (2006). *MacArthur–Bates communicative development inventories user's guide and technical manual* (2nd ed.). Brookes.

Fey, M. (2008). Thoughts on grammar intervention in AAC. *Perspectives on Augmentative and Alternative Communication, 17*(2), 43–49. https://doi.org/10.1044/aac17.2.43

Grogan-Johnson, S., Schmidt, A. M., Schenker, J., Alvares, R., Rowan, L. E., & Taylor, J. (2013). A comparison of speech sound intervention delivered by telepractice and side-by-side service delivery models. *Communication Disorders Quarterly, 34*(4), 210–220. https://doi.org/10.1177/1525740113484965

Hadley, P. A. (2014). Approaching early grammatical intervention from a sentence-focused framework. *Language, Speech, and Hearing Services in Schools, 45*(2), 110–116. https://doi.org/10.1044/2014_LSHSS-14-0017

Hadley, P. A., Rispoli, M. Holt, J. K., Papastratakos, T., Hsu, N., Kubalanza, M., . . . McKenna, M. (2017). Input subject diversity enhances early grammatical growth: Evidence from a parent-implemented intervention, *Language Learning and Development, 13*(1), 54–79. doi:10.1080/15475441.2016.1193020

Hall, N., Boisvert, M., Jellison, H., & Adrianopoulos, M. (2014). Language intervention via text-based tele-AAC: A case study comparing on-site and telepractice services. *Perspectives on Augmentative and Alternative Communication, 23*(1), 61–70. https://doi.org/10.1044/teles4.261

Hayes, L. E., & Traughber, M. C. (2021). Improving facilitation of student communication through observational feedback within a partner instruction model. *Language, Speech, and Hearing Services in Schools.* https://doi.org/10.1044/2020_LSHSS-20-00049

Hustad, K. C., Gorton, K., & Lee, J. (2010). Classification of speech and language profiles in 4-year-old children with cerebral palsy: A prospective preliminary study. *Journal of Speech, Language, and Hearing Research, 53*(6), 1496–1513. https://doi.org/10.1044/1092-4388(2010/09-0176)

Kasari, C., Kaiser, A., Goods, K., et al. (2014). Communication interventions for minimally verbal children with autism: A sequential multiple assignment randomized trial. *Journal of the American Academy of Child and Adolescent Psychiatry, 53*(6), 635–646. https://doi.org/10.1016/j.jaac.2014.01.019

Kent, R. D., & Vorperian, H. K. (2013). Speech impairment in down syndrome: A review. *Journal of Speech, Language, and Hearing Research, 56*(1), 178–210. https://doi.org/10.1044/1092-4388(2012/12-0148)

Kent-Walsh, J., Binger, C., & Buchanan, C. (2015). Teaching children who use augmentative and alternative communication to ask inverted yes/no questions using aided modeling. *American Journal of Speech-Language Pathology, 24*(2), 222–236. https://doi.org/10.1044/2015_AJSLP-14-0066

Kent-Walsh, J., Binger, C., & Hasham, Z. (2010). Effects of parent instruction on the symbolic communication of children using augmentative and alternative communication during storybook reading. *American Journal of Speech-Language Pathology, 19*, 97–107. https://doi.org/10.1044/1058-0360(2010/09-0014)

Kent-Walsh, J., Binger, C., & Malani, M. (2009). Teaching partners to support the communication skills of young children who use AAC: Lessons from the ImPAACT program. *Early Childhood Services, 4*(3), 155–170.

Kent-Walsh, J., Murza, K. A., Malani, M. D., & Binger, C. (2015). Effects of communication partner instruction on the communication of individuals using AAC: A meta-analysis. *AAC: Augmentative and Alternative Communication, 31*(4), 271–284. https://doi.org/10.3109/07434618.2015.1052153

Light, J., & McNaughton, D. (2014). Communicative competence for individuals who require augmentative and alternative communication: A new definition for a new era of communication? *AAC: Augmentative and Alternative Communication, 30*(1), 1–18. https://doi.org/10.3109/07434618.2014.885080

Lund, S. K., & Light, J. (2007). Long-term outcomes for individuals who use augmentative and alternative communication: Part III – Contributing factors. *AAC: Augmentative and Alternative Communication, 23*(4), 323–335. https://doi.org/10.1080/02656730701189123

McDonald, E., & Schultz, A. (1973). Communication boards for cerebral palsied children. *Journal of Speech and Hearing Disorders, 38,* 73–88.

O'Neill, T., Light, J., & Pope, L. (2018). Effects of interventions that include aided augmentative and alternative communication input on the communication of individuals with complex communication needs: A meta-analysis. *Journal of Speech, Language, and Hearing Research, 61*(7), 1743–1765. https://doi.org/10.1044/2018_JSLHR-L-17-0132

Rice, M. L., Smolik, F., Perpich, D., Thompson, T., Rytting, N., & Blossom, M. (2010). Mean length of utterance levels in 6-month intervals for children 3 to 9 years with and without language impairments. *Journal of Speech, Language, and Hearing Research, 53*(2), 333–349. https://doi.org/10.1044/1092-4388(2009/08-0183)

Romano, M., Kaiser, A., Lounds-Taylor, J., & Woods, J. (2020). Rates of prelinguistic communication and early symbol use in young children with down syndrome: Using a progress-monitoring tool to model growth. *American Journal of Speech-Language Pathology, 29*(1), 49–62. https://doi.org/10.1044/2019_AJSLP-19-0016

Romski, M., Sevcik, R. A., Adamson, L. B., Cheslock, M., Smith, A., Barker, R. M., . . . Bakeman, R. (2010). Randomized comparison of augmented and nonaugmented language interventions for toddlers with developmental delays and their parents. *Journal of Speech, Language, and Hearing Research, 53*(2), 350–364. https://doi.org/10.1044/1092-4388(2009/08-0156

Schlosser, R. W. (2002). On the importance of being earnest about treatment integrity. *Augmentative and Alternative Communication, 18,* 36–44. https://doi.org/10.1080/aac.18.1.36.44

Tonsing, K. M., Dada, S., & Alant, E. (2014). Teaching graphic symbol combinations to children with limited speech during shared story reading. *AAC: Augmentative and Alternative Communication, 30*(4), 279–297. https://doi.org/10.3109/07434618.2014.965846

5 Supporting Language and Literacy Learning for Children Who use AAC

Sally Clendon and Karen Erickson

Introduction

The link between language and literacy was established decades ago (Snow et al., 1999). Initially, oral language provides an important foundation for the later development of literacy (Snowling, 2005), but as literacy skills develop, the relationship becomes bidirectional, with improved literacy skills enhancing language skills and vice versa (e.g., Duff et al., 2015). This concurrent development of reading, writing, speaking (expressive language), and listening (receptive language) begins early in development (Koppenhaver et al., 1991; Teale & Sulzby, 1986). For some children with complex communication needs, understanding about literacy appears to precede clear expression of oral language understanding (Hanser & Erickson, 2007; Koppenhaver & Erickson, 2003). Regardless of the apparent order of development of language and literacy skills, the nature of their concurrent development is the basis of the rationale for comprehensive instruction that addresses all aspects of oral and written language.

The components of comprehensive literacy instruction differ depending on whether a student is emergent in their literacy learning or conventional. Comprehensive emergent literacy instruction involves daily opportunities for children to engage with text, to build their communication and language skills in authentic and meaningful literacy-related activities and interactions, and to develop specific emergent literacy skills recognised as critical for literacy success (e.g., alphabet knowledge, phonological awareness, print concept knowledge). A classroom programme supporting emergent literacy skills includes activities such as shared reading and writing, independent reading and writing, and working with letters and sounds (Erickson & Koppenhaver, 2020).

Comprehensive conventional literacy instruction focuses on skills needed to become independent, effective readers and writers whereby children can read texts silently with comprehension, write texts that can be read and understood by others, and have the decoding, spelling, and word identification abilities needed to read, write, and communicate with success. A classroom programme to develop conventional literacy skills includes daily instruction in at least four key areas: reading comprehension, word study, self-directed reading, and writing (Erickson & Koppenhaver, 2020).

DOI: 10.4324/9781003106739-5

In addition to providing access to a comprehensive literacy programme, it is important that educational teams understand children's literacy profiles. This can assist with prioritising any additional input and support, and it can influence decision making regarding team members' contributions to the literacy programme (Clendon et al., 2021; Erickson et al., 2016). With language and literacy so entwined, team members can integrate their individual expertise collaboratively to optimise literacy outcomes as illustrated in the case that follows.

Case Report

Background Information

Jamie (aged 7 years, 2 months) attended his local school where he was included in a classroom with 25 peers. He had a supportive team, which included his family (mum, dad, older brother), his teacher, a classroom teaching assistant, the school learning support coordinator, and his speech-language therapist (SLT). Jamie enjoyed physical activity, playing soccer, basketball, and riding his bike. At school he was involved in a variety of clubs and activities, and liked most aspects of the classroom programme, particularly maths, inquiry (especially science topics), shared reading, and visits to the school library where he was drawn to nonfiction books about sports, animals, and science. He had two best friends in his classroom.

Presenting Concerns

Jamie had a genetic syndrome that has resulted in childhood apraxia of speech. He had motor difficulties that became evident when he started school and experienced difficulties with handwriting. He had speech-language therapy from the age of 18 months, focused on speech sound development and the implementation of AAC. Initially, Jamie used keyword signs and a communication board with core and fringe vocabulary. At age four, he started using a comprehensive communication app on an iPad.

Jamie's teacher Rob had five years' teaching experience. Jamie was the first student with complex communication needs that he had taught. He wanted to include Jamie as much as possible in class and invested significant time getting to know Jamie and his AAC system. Rob had observed Jamie in his previous year's class. He noted that Jamie was an active participant in the literacy program, but the classroom teaching assistant, Sophie, typically guided him through each activity. For example, when the children were writing, Sophie stretched out each word, providing phoneme-by-phoneme support for each word he wrote. Rob understood that this was likely interfering with Jamie's independence in decoding and spelling (Gonzalez-Frey & Ehri, 2020). When the children were reading silently, Sophie read the text aloud to Jamie. Rob knew that Jamie benefitted from Sophie's reading, but he also knew that children learn many important skills during independent silent reading (Deacon et al., 2019). At

Jamie's recent progress meeting, Rob asked the team for support in assessing Jamie's literacy skills and interpreting results to guide instructional decisions to facilitate more independent reading and writing.

Clinical Findings

The team assessed Jamie's language and literacy skills using a comprehensive battery of assessments (see Table 5.1).

Receptive Language

Jamie obtained a standard score of 97 on the Peabody Picture Vocabulary Test (PPVT-5; Dunn, 2018) and 83 on the Test for Reception of Grammar (TROG-2; Bishop, 2003). He had difficulty understanding complex sentences such as "The pencil is not only long but also red". When asked to listen to three progressively more complex passages from the Basic Reading Inventory (BRI; Johns et al., 2016), Jamie responded with 100% and 90% accuracy to the first and second passages respectively, but only 63% accuracy to the third, indicating that he understood text at the second-grade level but his comprehension started to break down with more complex texts.

Expressive Language

On the Expressive One Word Picture Vocabulary Test (EOWPVT-4; Martin, & Brownell, 2011), Jamie obtained a standard score of 70 using his AAC system. An analysis of language samples revealed that Jamie was at Phase 3 of the Graphic Symbol Utterance and Sentence Development Framework (Binger et al., 2020). He was able to use three-part clause structures (e.g., *HE GO PARTY, SHE JUMP HIGH*), usually with correct word order, and a range of word classes (e.g., nouns, verbs, adjectives, prepositions). He frequently omitted phrasal elements (e.g., copula verb, auxiliaries, determiners) and inflectional morphemes (e.g., plural, past tense). His mean length of utterance in symbols (MLUSym) was 3.4.

Early Literacy

Jamie responded correctly to all items on the Concepts about Print assessment (Clay, 2000). On the Letter-Sound Identification probe (Erickson et al., 2005), he identified all upper- and lower-case letters and all letter-sounds, with the exception of upper and lower case 'G' and lower case 'q'. His scores on the Rhyme Detection and Phoneme Identity probes (Gillon, 2005) were 8/10 and 10/10, respectively. Jamie scored 4/42 on the Invented Spelling measure (Lombardino et al., 2010). He was able to represent three initial phonemes and one final sound (M for *mail*, F for *feet*, and DS for *dress*). On the Word Identification measure (Lombardino et al., 2010), Jamie identified 6/10 basal or sight words, and 3/10 decodable words. He wrote his name accurately and scored 8 on Bingham et al.'s (2017) 8-point scale. Two writing samples were obtained;

Table 5.1 Language and Literacy Assessment Battery

Area of Assessment	Test/Task	Type of Test/Scoring	Notes
Receptive Language			
Single–Word Vocabulary	Peabody Picture Vocabulary Test (PPVT-5; Dunn, 2018) vocabulary	Standardized norm-referenced test	No adaptations required
Sentence-Level Comprehension	Test for Reception of Grammar – Version 2 (TROG-2, Bishop, 2003)	Standardized norm-referenced test	Test discontinued after three failed sections
Narrative-Level Comprehension	Assessed using an End of Kindergarten (End-K), Beginning Grade 1 (Beg-1), and Middle Grade 1 (Mid-1) passage from the Basic Reading Inventory (BRI, Johns et al., 2016)	Informal; maximum score of 9 for End-K, 10 for Beg-1, and 16 for Mid-1	Modified with comprehension questions adapted for multichoice and yes/no responses (Center for Literacy and Disability Studies, 2016)
Expressive Language			
Single–Word Vocabulary	Expressive One Word Vocabulary Test (EOWPVT-4, Brownell, 2010)	Standardized norm-referenced test	Checked words being assessed were available in AAC system prior to administration
Utterance and Sentence Complexity	Language samples obtained at home and school	Informal	Analysed using suggested measures by Binger et al. (2020) describing the Graphic Symbol Utterance and Sentence Development Framework
Early Literacy			
Print Concept Knowledge	Marie Clay's (2000) Concepts about Print assessment with specially modified text	Informal; maximum score of 14	Modified as per Erickson et al. (2005) so as not to require a spoken response
Letter Name Knowledge and Letter Sound Knowledge	Letter-Sound Identification probe (Erickson et al., 2005) – asked to point to a target letter or sound from a field of six	Informal; maximum score of 52 for Letter Name Knowledge and 52 for Letter Sound Knowledge	Letters arranged on A4 sheets of paper; both upper case and lower case letters presented

(Continued)

Table 5.1 (Continued)

Area of Assessment	Test/Task	Type of Test/Scoring	Notes
Name Writing	Assessed and scored using the procedure outlined in Bingham et al. (2017) – asked to write name	Informal; 8-point scale: 0 = refusal; 1 = scribbling; 2 = drawing as writing; 3 = scribble writing; 4 = letter-like shapes; 5 = letters and letter-like shapes; 6 = partial word/name; 7 = all letters in name, incorrect order; 8 = correct	Provided with pencil and blank piece of paper
Phonological Awareness	Rhyme Detection and Phoneme Matching Probes (Gillon, 2005)	Informal; maximum score of 10 for each probe	No adaptations required
Invented Spelling	Assessed using the Phoneme Awareness task from the Early Reading Screening Inventory (ERSI; Lombardino et al., 1999) – asked to spell 12 words	Informal; one point for each phoneme represented within each word; maximum score of 42	Completed using alphabet page in AAC system
Word identification	Assessed using the Word Recognition task from the ERSI (Lombardino et al., 1999) – one list of 10 sight words and one list of 10 decodable words	Informal; maximum score of 10 for each wordlist	Modified as per Erickson et al. (2005); asked to select target word from a field of four, which included three distracter words that began with the same letter and were of similar length
Writing	Writing samples obtained and scored using the Developmental Writing Scale (Sturm et al., 2012)	Informal; maximum score of 14	First sample completed using pencil; second sample completed using alphabet page in AAC system

one with a pencil, and one using the alphabet page in his AAC system. The samples were evaluated using the Developmental Writing Scale (Sturm et al., 2012) and placed at Level 4 (letter strings grouped in words) with the pencil, and Level 5 (one intelligible word) with the AAC system.

Summary, Interpretation, and Initial Hypothesis

The language and literacy assessments showed that Jamie had relatively strong receptive language skills. His expressive language needs included expanding vocabulary and sentence complexity, particularly through the inclusion of key phrasal elements and inflectional morphemes. The literacy assessments revealed strengths in early literacy skills, including letter-sound knowledge and phonological awareness. The Invented Spelling, Word Identification, and Writing assessments indicated that he was in the early stages of applying his phonological knowledge to reading and writing.

Diagnostic Intervention

Jamie's classroom literacy programme included daily reading comprehension instruction, word study, self-directed reading, and writing. This programme would foster the skills necessary to develop conventional literacy; however, some components of the programme required differentiation to optimise Jamie's success. Jamie's teacher and broader educational team considered the key conditions for learning (Erickson & Koppenhaver, 2020). They aimed to have high expectations for Jamie, continue to develop his language skills using his AAC system, provide repetition with variety to keep learning interesting, maximise Jamie's cognitive engagement and cognitive clarity, and build Jamie's self-efficacy so he felt empowered to take risks in his learning. Rob also identified strategies for increasing Jamie's independence in reading and writing.

Application of Letter-Sound Knowledge

Jamie needed support to apply his letter-sound knowledge. Such support can be through explicit and systematic word instruction, as well as frequent writing opportunities. It was agreed that word instruction would focus on building Jamie's decoding, spelling, and word identification skills. This would ensure he could build the automaticity he needed to read and spell high frequency words with ease, freeing up his cognitive resources so that he could focus on reading for meaning. In addition, instruction targeted the decoding skills needed to read and spell words not directly taught. Two instructional approaches that work well for children with complex communication needs are Making Words (see Table 5.2), a spelling-based approach, and Onset-Rime instruction, an analogy-based approach (both described in detail in Erickson & Koppenhaver, 2020). Neither approach requires children to respond orally, yet both provide teachers with moment-to-moment feedback regarding students' understanding of letters and letter-sounds in reading and spelling words. They also minimise the meta-cognitive demands of learning to read words. For example, Onset-Rime instruction focuses on supporting children to learn keywords (e.g., *at*) and then to use these keywords to read and spell other words (e.g., *hat, cat, rat, flat*). This approach is less cognitively demanding than approaches that require children to learn and apply a series of rules (Erickson & Koppenhaver, 2020).

Making Words lessons (Cunningham & Hall, 2008) target the development of decoding skills. They teach students to look for spelling patterns in words and recognise the differences that result when a single letter is changed. The lessons get systematically more challenging.

Lesson Format

Each student needs their own set of letters. Lessons have four parts, as shown in Table 5.2 after the text Lessons have four parts.

Table 5.2 Making Words Overview

1. Name the letters and their sounds	• Hand out the letters that will be used in the lesson (e.g., *a, b, m, n, t*) one at a time. As you pass out each letter, ask the students to think of a word that starts with that letter. For example: *This letter is **M**. M represents the /m/ sound. Can you think of a word that starts with /m/?*
2. Make words with the letters	• Guide the students in making the words included in the lesson. Ensure that there are only minimal changes from one word to the next. For example, in the lesson with the letters above, you might ask them to make the words **a**, **an**, **at**, **bat**, **mat**, **man**, **ban**, and **tan**
	• As you present each word, put it into a sentence. For example:
	o *Take one letter and make **a**. I am **a** teacher*
	o *Add a letter to **a** and you can spell **an**. I want **an** apple*
	o *Take the **n** away and add a different letter to make **at**. We are **at** school*
	• Encourage the students to use their letters to make each word
	• After they have made their attempt, show them the correctly spelled word, and have them compare their spelling letter by letter and make corrections if necessary.
	• Provide instructional feedback. For example, if you ask the students to make the word ***bat*** and they make ***nat***, you can say: *This word says **nat**. We are trying to make **bat**. Let me show you how I make **bat**. Can you make your word look like mine?*
	• As the words are made, write them in a list so that the students can see the words changing as you go through the lesson.
3. Sort the words that you have made	• Start by reading through the lists of all the words that were made.
	• Then ask the students to sort the words into columns according to different features. For example, you might ask them to sort according to the number of letters within the word, or the letter that the words start with, or the vowels within the words.
4. Transfer	• Ask the students to transfer or apply their learning from the lesson to spell words that weren't directly taught. For example, in the lesson above, you might ask the students to spell **rat** and **cat** in the transfer step.

Source: Cunningham, P. M., & Hall, D. P. (2008). *Making words first grade: 100 hands-on lessons for phonemic awareness, phonics, and spelling.* Pearson.

Jamie also needed explicit teaching to apply his decoding and word identification skills to spelling. A word wall (see Erickson & Koppenhaver, 2020 and Appendix 5.1) can support the spelling of high frequency words and the use of keywords to spell words that share the same spelling pattern. Rather than providing Jamie with phoneme-by-phoneme support for spelling, his teaching assistant, Sophie, could refer to the word wall: "You want to spell *bike*? There's a word on your word wall that will help you with that. It's one of your keywords". Jamie also needed support to apply his decoding skills to his spelling. This instruction involved encouraging him to make independent spelling attempts for words he didn't yet know how to spell, representing the sounds that he could hear in words, for example "BSKTBL" for *basketball*. Modelling was important for encouraging Jamie not to stick only to the words he already knew how to spell.

Rob already had a word wall in the classroom and developed a plan to embed the keyword approach within this. The Making Words lessons were potentially beneficial for a group of students who all needed additional support. He worked with Sophie to plan how they would both model and support Jamie with his word reading and spelling across the day. Jamie's SLT, Aimee, offered to lead one of the Making Words lessons each week, and to work with Rob in monitoring Jamie's progress.

Expressive Language Intervention

Jamie's assessment indicated he needed explicit support to build expressive vocabulary and sentence complexity. Aimee discussed the importance of providing aided language input, being responsive communication partners, and looking for opportunities to expand Jamie's expressive language. Aimee used the language samples collated for the literacy assessment to identify specific language structures to teach (e.g., copular verb, auxiliaries) and targeted these structures through focused stimulation (Binger et al., 2011; Solomon-Rice & Soto, 2014) in her sessions with Jamie.

With coaching support from Aimee, Rob started to work on optimising the shared readings that were part of his classroom literacy programme. Aimee demonstrated the CROWD in the CAR framework (see Clendon et al., 2014; Erickson & Koppenhaver, 2020 and Appendix 5.2), and Rob and Sophie learned to facilitate interaction, use wait time, and employ a variety of prompts to elicit language from Jamie and other students. In shared reading, adults read and scaffold interactions across a story. In contrast, in comprehension instruction, children are supported to independently read texts of increasing length and complexity. Activation of background knowledge is a critical element of reading comprehension, as children need to create a cognitive representation by merging the information in the text with relevant background knowledge (Castles et al., 2018). Rob was keen to move Jamie into comprehension instruction (alongside ongoing shared reading) before the end of the school year and together with Aimee they developed a plan to support Jamie to make connections with existing background knowledge and read for a purpose such as to make a prediction or organise key information from the text (see Erickson & Koppenhaver, 2020).

Word knowledge is fundamental to language comprehension and an essential part of literacy (Beck & McKeown, 2007; National Research Council, 1998; Roskos et al., 2008). Rob combined direct vocabulary instruction with indirect experiences across the curriculum (Marulis & Neuman, 2010) to extend Jamie's vocabulary. Effective vocabulary instruction goes beyond teaching definitions to an emphasis on multiple word meanings, understanding situations of use, and making associations between new and known words (Duff, 2019; Duff et al., 2015; McKeown, 2019). Rob focused on strategically connecting new words that Jamie encountered in texts and other curriculum areas to words that were familiar to him. Until Jamie learned to write to express his thoughts, he would be limited by the words in his AAC system. Thus, he benefitted greatly from learning to use the words in his system to express understandings of new words and associated concepts (Erickson, 2003; Erickson & Koppenhaver, 2020; Geist & Erickson, 2021; Van Tatenhove, 2009).

The connections Jamie made between new and known words helped build the deep understandings that would make it possible for him to interpret the meaning of a word encountered in a new context (Beck et al., 2013; Erickson & Koppenhaver, 2020; Perfetti, 2007). This approach to using known words to communicate about new words in AAC has been described as a form of circumlocution (Erickson, 2003), with one systematic approach known as *descriptive teaching* (Van Tatenhove, 2009; Witkowski & Baker, 2012). Rob wanted Jamie to think flexibly about words on a conceptual level, while helping him learn to communicate understanding of a broad range of vocabulary without programming hundreds of new words into Jamie's AAC system (Geist & Erickson, 2021).

To select target vocabulary, Rob used Beck and colleagues' (Beck et al., 2008, 2013) three tiers framework. Jamie's assessment confirmed that he has learned to understand and use words classified as Tier 1 (i.e., common words that the majority of children learn through everyday interactions, often before they enter school). Rob focused on Tier 2 words – those words that have the highest utility, appear across a variety of curriculum contexts, and will build success across oral and written language tasks (Erickson & Koppenhaver, 2020; McKeown, 2019). Rob included a few Tier 3 words (e.g., amendment, equator) that are domain-specific and rare (Beck et al., 2013) and ensured that Tier 3 words appeared frequently enough that Jamie could learn their meaning and use, while increasing his ability to use the words available on his AAC system to talk about them (e.g., describe amendment as *make little change* or *add more*).

Intervention Progress

Jamie's team understood the need to monitor progress in order to reflect on their instructional decisions. They committed to minimizing the time they spent assessing Jamie and instead focused on analysing the product of his work.

Writing Sample Analysis

Jamie's teacher, Rob, engaged his students in writing across the curriculum. These writing products enabled him to track Jamie's writing progress. Rob selected at least one writing sample every two weeks to analyse using *The Developmental Writing Scale* (see Sturm et al., 2012). He also analysed the writing samples to track Jamie's progress in spelling, as well as vocabulary and language use. For example, the words that Jamie spelled correctly and incorrectly in his writing revealed important information about his application of letter-sound knowledge. Rob tracked the percentage of phonemes that Jamie represented correctly, and the high frequency words that he spelled correctly. This combination provided vital information regarding the relative success of the decoding, spelling, and word identification instruction provided and informed next steps in instruction. Rob also tracked the number of different words, as well as the length of t-units (Scott, 2020) and number of different ideas that Jamie included in each writing sample.

Maze Assessment

Rob's practice was to listen to his students read aloud and evaluate comprehension by asking them to summarize what they had read. This approach wasn't possible with Jamie, but Rob was also reticent to rely entirely on multiple choice questions to track comprehension of connected text. Jamie's SLT, Aimee, explained that reading with *maze* can be used to monitor progress in reading (Graney et al., 2010; Guthrie, 1973). Together, Rob and Aimee created maze passages using texts that Rob planned to use with Jamie. They extracted passages of 100 to 125 words in length. They left the first two sentences intact, and then, beginning with the fifth word of the third sentence, they deleted every fifth word and replaced it with a blank. For each blank, they prepared three answer options: (1) the original word, (2) a word that is the same part of speech as the original word, and (3) another word from the text that is structurally similar to the target word.

Following the guidelines offered by Erickson et al. (2016), they asked Jamie to complete repeated reading with maze every other week. First, they asked Jamie to complete the prepared maze task and confirmed that he scored 50% or higher to ensure that the text was at an appropriate level. Then, Jamie practiced with the original text three or four times before repeating the maze task. If he then scored in the range of 80% correct, he was asked to read the text three or four more times and complete the maze passage one more time to confirm that he had reached an accuracy of 90% or higher. If Jamie did not score in the range of 80%, they discontinued and found an easier text. Importantly, these were all tasks that Jamie could complete on his own in school or at home, helping the team to gauge the complexity of the text they selected for Jamie throughout the curriculum.

Language Sample Analysis

The SLT, Aimee, analysed Jamie's writing samples with Rob to monitor Jamie's development of vocabulary and sentence structure. In addition, Aimee collected language samples once each school term and analysed these using key measures from the Graphic Symbol Utterance and Sentence Development Framework (Binger et al., 2020). Rob and Aimee also introduced a notebook for the team to capture examples of Jamie's language as they occurred across the day (e.g., if Jamie demonstrated understanding of a new Tier 2 word during shared reading by using his AAC system to describe the new word).

Outcomes

Rob enjoyed the opportunity to spend the rest of the year with Jamie. The results of the assessment combined with the work the team completed to interpret the results and plan an instructional program for Jamie gave him confidence that teaching a student with complex communication needs could be enriching and successful.

Reflections and Considerations

Five years on and Jamie is now 12 years of age. Reflecting back, the year in Rob's class laid a critical foundation for success in Jamie's language and literacy development. Several factors contributed to this success, including the enthusiasm with which Rob and the broader team embraced the key conditions of learning, such as having high expectations, developing Jamie's language using his AAC system, and building his self-efficacy. Another key factor was the provision of a comprehensive classroom literacy programme alongside explicit teaching and targeted support in key areas. Language and literacy assessment was a critical part of this process – identifying Jamie's strengths and needs, determining a plan for instruction, establishing different team member's contributions, and monitoring Jamie's progress. Rob and Aimee built a strong collaborative relationship and worked together to optimise Jamie's success and facilitate his transition into the following school year. Jamie is now an academically competitive student who can use his literacy skills for a range of purposes, including accessing and engaging with the curriculum, networking socially with his friends, and supporting his face-to-face communication. He moves independently through the school, seeks support when needed, and thrives as a member of his classroom and broader school community.

References

Beck, I. L., & McKeown, M. G. (2007). Increasing young low-income children's oral vocabulary repertoires through rich and focused instruction. *Elementary School Journal*, *107*, 251–271. https://doi.org/10.1086/511706

Beck, I. L., McKeown, M. G., & Kucan, L. (2008). *Creating robust vocabulary: Frequently asked questions and extended examples.* Guilford Publications.

Beck, I. L., McKeown, M. G., & Kucan, L. (2013). *Bringing words to life: Robust vocabulary instruction.* Guilford Publications.

Binger, C., Kent-Walsh, J., Harrington, N., & Hollerback, Q. (2020). Tracking early sentence-building progress in graphic symbol communication. *Language, Speech, and Hearing Services in Schools, 51,* 317–328. https://doi.org/10.1044/2019_LSHSS-19-00065

Binger, C., Maguire-Marshall, M., & Kent-Walsh, J. (2011). Using aided AAC models, recasts, and contrastive targets to teach grammatical morphemes to children who use AAC. *Journal of Speech, Language and Hearing Research, 54,* 160–176. https://doi.org/10.1044/1092-4388(2010/09-0163)

Bingham, G. E., Quinn, M. F., & Gerde, H. K. (2017). Examining early childhood teachers' writing practices: Associations between pedagogical supports and children's writing skills. *Early Childhood Research Quarterly, 39,* 35–46. https://doi.org/10.1016/j.ecresq.2017.01.002

Bishop, D. V. M. (2003). *Test for the reception of grammar: TROG-2.* Pearson.

Brownell, R. (2010). *Expressive one word vocabulary test: EOWPVT-4.* Pearson.

Castles, A., Rastle, K., & Nation, K. (2018). Ending the reading wards: Reading acquisition from novice to expert. *Psychological Science in the Public Interest, 19,* 5–51. https://doi:10.1177/1529100618772271

Center for Literacy and Disability Studies. (2016). *Modified basic reading inventory* [Unpublished assessment]. University of North Carolina at Chapel Hill.

Clay, M. M. (2000). *Concepts about print: What have children learned about the way we print language?* Heinemann.

Clendon, S., Erickson, K. A., van Rensburg, R., & Amm, J. (2014). Shared storybook reading: An authentic context for developing literacy, language, and communication skills. *Perspectives on Augmentative and Alternative Communication, 23*(4), 182–191. https://pubs.asha.org/doi/10.1044/aac23.4.182

Clendon, S., Paynter, J., Walker, S., Bowen, R., & Westerveld, M. (2021). Emergent literacy assessment in children with autism spectrum disorder who have limited verbal communication needs: A tutorial. *Language, Speech, and Hearing Services in the Schools, 52,* 165–180. https://doi.org/10.1044/2020_LSHSS-20-00030

Deacon, S. H., Mimeau, C., Chung, S. C., & Chen, X. (2019). Young readers' skill in learning spellings and meanings of words during independent reading. *Journal of Experimental Child Psychology, 181,* 56–74. https://doi-org.libproxy.lib.unc.edu/10.1016/j.jecp.2018.12.007

Duff, D. (2019). The effect of vocabulary intervention on text comprehension: Who benefits? *Language, Speech, and Hearing Services in Schools, 50,* 562–578. https://doi.org/10.1044/2019_LSHSS-VOIA-18-0001

Duff, D., Tomblin, J. B., & Catts, H. (2015). The influence of reading on vocabulary growth: A case for a Matthew effect. *Journal of Speech Language and Hearing Research, 58*(3), 853–864. https://doi.org/10.1044/2015_JSLHR-L-13-0310

Dunn, D. M. (2018). *Peabody picture vocabulary test – 5: PPVT-5.* Pearson.

Erickson, K. A. (2003). Reading comprehension in AAC. *ASHA Leader, 8*(12), 6–9. https://doi.org/10.1044/leader.FTR1.08122003.6

Erickson, K. A., Clendon, S., Abraham, L., Roy, V., & Van de Carr, H. (2005). Toward positive literacy outcomes for students with significant developmental disabilities. *Assistive Technology Outcomes and Benefits, 2*(1), 45–54.

Erickson, K. A., & Koppenhaver, D. A. (2020). *Comprehensive literacy for all: Teaching students with significant disabilities to read and write.* Brookes.

Erickson, K. A., Koppenhaver, D. A., & Cunningham, J. W. (2016). Balanced reading intervention in augmentative communication. In R. McCauley, M. Fey, & R. Gillam (Eds.), *Treatment of language disorders in children* (2nd ed., pp. 275–308). Brookes.

Geist, L., & Erickson, K. (2021). Robust receptive vocabulary instruction for students with significant cognitive disabilities who use AAC. *Teaching Exceptional Children.* https://doi.org/10.1177%2F00400599211018836

Gillon, G. (2005). *Phonological awareness probes.* www.canterbury.ac.nz/education-and-health/research/phonological-awareness-resources

Gonzalez-Frey, S. M., & Ehri, L. (2020). Connected phonation is more effective than segmented phonation for teaching beginning readers to decode unfamiliar words. *Scientific Studies of Reading.* https://doi.org/10.1080/10888438.2020.1776290

Graney, S. B., Martínez, R. S., Missall, K. N., & Aricak, O. T. (2010). Universal screening of reading in late elementary school: R-CBM versus CBM Maze. *Remedial and Special Education, 31,* 368–377. https://doi.org/10.1177/0741932509338371

Guthrie, J. T. (1973). Reading comprehension and syntactic responses in good and poor readers. *Journal of Educational Psychology, 65,* 294–300. https://doi:10.1037/h0035643

Hanser, G., & Erickson, K. (2007). Integrated word identification and communication instruction for students with complex communication needs: Preliminary results. *Focus on Autism and Developmental Disabilities, 22*(4), 268–278. https://doi.org/10.1177/10883576070220040901

Johns, J., Johns, B., & Elish Piper, L. (2016). *Basic reading inventory: Kindergarten through grade twelve and early literacy assessments* (12th ed.) [assessment]. Kendall Hunt.

Koppenhaver, D., Coleman, P., Kalman, S., & Yoder, D. (1991). The implications of emergent literacy research for children with developmental disabilities. *American Journal of Speech-Language Pathology: A Journal of Clinical Practice, 1*(1), 38–44. https://doi.org/10.1044/1058-0360.0101.38

Koppenhaver, D., & Erickson, K. (2003). Natural emergent literacy supports for preschoolers with autism and severe communication impairments. *Topics in Language Disorders, 23*(4), 283–292. https://doi.org/10.1097/00011363-200310000-00004

Lombardino, L. J., Morris, D., Mercado, L., DeFillipo, F., Sarisky, C., & Montgomery, C. (1999). The early reading screening instrument: A method for identifying kindergarteners at risk for learning to read. *International Journal of Language and Communication Disorders, 34*(2), 135–150. https://doi.org/10.1080/136828299247478

Martin, N. A., & Brownell, R. (2011). *EOWPVT-4: Expressive one-word picture vocabulary test* (4th ed.) [assessment]. Pro-ed.

Marulis, L. M., & Neuman, S. B. (2010). The effects of vocabulary intervention on young children's word learning: A meta-analysis. *Review of Educational Research, 80*(3), 300–335. https://doi.org/10.3102/0034654310377087

McKeown, M. (2019). Effective vocabulary instruction fosters knowing words, using words, and understanding how words work. *Language, Speech, and Hearing Services in Schools, 50,* 466–476. https://doi.org/10.1044/2019_LSHSS-VOIA-18-0126

National Research Council. (1998). *Preventing reading difficulties in young children.* The National Academies Press. https://doi.org/10.17226/6023

Perfetti, C. A. (2007). Reading ability: Lexical quality to comprehension. *Scientific Studies of Reading, 11,* 357–383. https://doi.org/10.1080/10888430701530730

Roskos, K., Ergul, C., Bryan, T., Burstein, K., Christie, J., & Han, M. (2008). Who's learning what words and how fast: Preschoolers' vocabulary growth in an early literacy program. *Journal of Research in Childhood Education, 22,* 49–63. https://doi.org/10.1080/02568540809594627

Scott, C. M. (2020). Language sample analysis of writing in children and adolescents. *Topics in Language Disorders, 40*(2), 202–220. https://doi.org/10.1097/TLD.0000000000000213

Snow, C., Scarborough, H., & Burns, M. (1999). What speech-language pathologists need to know about early reading. *Topics in Language Disorders, 20*, 48–58. https://doi.org/10.1097/00011363-199911000-00006

Snowling, M. (2005). Phonological processing and developmental dyslexia. *Journal of Research in Reading, 18*(2), 132–138. https://doi.org/10.1111/j.1467-9817.1995.tb00079.x

Solomon-Rice, P. L., & Soto, G. (2014). Facilitating vocabulary in toddlers using AAC: A preliminary study comparing focused stimulation and augmented input. *Communication Disorders Quarterly, 35*(4), 204–215. https://doi.org/10.1177/1525740114522856

Sturm, J., Cali, K., Nelson, N., & Staskowsi, M. (2012). The developmental writing scale: A new progress monitoring tool for beginning writers. *Topics in Language Disorders, 32*(4), 287–318. http://dx.doi.org/10.1097/TLD.0b013e318272159e

Teale, W., & Sulzby, E. (1986). *Emergent literacy: Writing and reading.* Ablex.

Van Tatenhove, G. (2009). Building language competence with students using AAC devices: Six challenges. *Perspectives on Augmentative and Alternative Communication, 18*(2), 38–47. https://pubs.asha.org/doi/abs/10.1044/aac18.2.38

Witkowski, D., & Baker, B. (2012). Addressing the content vocabulary with core: Theory and practice for non-literate or emerging literate students. *Perspectives on Augmentative and Alternative Communication, 21*, 74–81. https://pubs.asha.org/doi/pdf/10.1044/aac21.3.74

Appendix 5.1

Word Wall Overview

Word Wall (Cunningham, 2016) is used to teach words that we want students to be able to read and spell with automaticity. Words are introduced gradually across the school year. Students are provided with daily opportunities to interact with the Word Wall. This includes 15–20 minutes of explicit Word Wall teaching. In addition, the Word Wall is referred to across the day whenever students are reading and spelling.

Selecting Words for the Word Wall

The words on the Word Wall are selected from two primary sources:

1. ***Keywords:*** These are a particularly important feature of Word Wall. The starting point for determining these is Wylie and Durrell's (1970) list of the 37 most common rimes in written English. For each rime pattern, one keyword is selected to go on the Word Wall to represent that pattern, for example, *make* may be selected to go on the Word Wall to represent the –ake pattern.
2. ***Other High Frequency Words:*** that appear across texts, e.g., *I, have, the.*

A small number of other words might be selected that have high utility (e.g., school name, favourite TV show) (Table A5.1).

Table A5.1 Thirty-seven Most Common Rimes in Written English (Wylie and Durrell, 1970)

–ack	–ail	–ain	–ake	–ale	–ame	–an
–ank	–ap	–ash	–at	–ate	–aw	–ay
–eat	–ell	–est	–ice	–ick	–ide	–ight
–ill	–in	–ine	–ing	–ink	–ip	–it
–ock	–oke	–op	–ore	–ot	–uck	–ug
–ump	–unk					

Setting up a Word Wall

The Word Wall is set up with 26 letters of the alphabet as headers. Below each letter, there needs to be sufficient space to display words in a font size large enough that the students can see the words easily. If insufficient wall space is available, or students need to be able to take their Word Wall with them to different classrooms, then a portable word wall may be more suitable.

New words added to the Word Wall are put directly under the other words that are already on the Word Wall under that letter. *Do not rearrange* the words within each letter so that they are in alphabetical order. Word Wall is about supporting students to build automaticity. Moving words around interrupts this process.

When *adding a keyword to the Word Wall, put a star next to it* so students learn that these are the words that they can use to help them to read and spell other words.

Teaching Word Wall

Up to five new words are added to the Word Wall each week. On Monday, when the new words are introduced, teach the meaning of the words, use them in sentences, find them in the students' AAC systems, and clap, chant, and write them letter by letter using a pencil, keyboard, or alphabet display. Encourage children who use AAC to chant the words subvocally.

On the remaining days of the week, complete short activities using the new words and previously introduced words on the Word Wall. There are thousands of ideas for Word Wall activities on the internet.

Whenever the students are reading or spelling across the day, refer them back to the Word Wall – "*There's a word on the Word Wall that might help you with that . . .*", "*it's one of your keywords*".

Appendix 5.2
CROWD in the CAR Overview

This strategy was developed by Dr. Patsy Pierce and is part of the Tar Heel Shared Reader programme (http://sharedreader.org) at the Center for Literacy and Disability Studies at the University of North Carolina at Chapel Hill (www.med.unc.edu/ahs/cld). It combines two evidence-based approaches used to support communication partners to interact more effectively during shared storybook reading.

The first approach is the **CAR** (adapted from Notari-Syverson et al., 2002): **C**omment and wait, **A**sk for participation and wait, and **R**espond by adding a little more.

The second approach is the **CROWD** (Whitehurst et al., 1994), which consists of five different language prompts that adults cycle through while reading with children: **C**ompletion, **R**ecall, **O**pen-ended, **W**h- questions, and **D**istancing.

- **Completion** prompts require children to "fill-in" a word left out by the reader; for example, "the dog is _____"
- **Recall** prompts or questions ask children to recall key elements of a story.
- **Open-ended** questions require children to talk about the story in their own words.
- **Wh- questions** elicit responses to "who", "what", "where", "when", or "why" questions.
- **Distancing** prompts or questions help children to relate what is happening in the book to their own experiences.

If children respond to the comment (C) made by the adult in the first step of the CAR, then the adult responds and extends the interaction. If children don't respond to the comment (C), then the adult can use the CROWD prompts to ask children to participate during the ask (A) step of the CAR. Children who are not yet using their AAC system expressively will need others to model all three steps of the CAR.

Getting Started

When first getting started, it can help to prepare for shared reading interactions by putting sticky notes on pages in the story. Write down the Comment you will make initially (e.g., OH NO, LOOK at the elephant), and also the CROWD prompt that you will use if needed (e.g., SHE is is FEELing _____). Underline the words that you plan to model on the child's AAC system.

Other Considerations

1. Provide repetition with variety. Read the same book across a week but stop on different pages.
2. Provide lots of wait time.
3. Attribute meaning to all attempts to communicate and to any messages expressed.
4. Refer to letters when you see them on a page (e.g., letters in the children's names).
5. Point out rhyming words and alliteration.
6. Point out print concepts, e.g., title page, where to begin reading.
7. Teach new vocabulary by connecting it to vocabulary in the child's AAC system, for example, "squillions of books – squillions – that means *A LOT*".

References

Cunningham, P. M. (2016). *Phonics they use: Words for reading and spelling* (7th ed.). Pearson.

Notari-Syverson, A., Maddox, M., Lim, Y. S., & Cole, K. (2002). *Language is the key: A program for building language and literacy*. Washington Research Institute.

Whitehurst, G. J., Arnold, D. S., Epstein, J. N., Angell, A. L., Smith, M., & Fischel, J. E. (1994). A picture book reading intervention in day care and home for children from low-income families. *Developmental Psychology, 30*, 679–689.

Wylie, R., & Durrell, D. (1970). Teaching vowels through phonograms. *Elementary English, 47*(6), 787–791.

6 Using AAC Principles to Guide Language Instruction for Autistic Individuals

A Case Report

Leigh Anne White, Maria Galassi, Loren F. McMahon, Anna A. Allen, Ralf W. Schlosser, Suzanne Flynn, Christina Yu and Howard C. Shane

Introduction

One in 54 children aged eight years in the United States currently meets the diagnostic criteria for autism spectrum disorder (ASD) (Maenner et al., 2020). The diagnostic criteria for ASD include persistent deficits in social communication and restricted or repetitive patterns of behavior, interests, or activities (American Psychiatric Association, 2013). Neither receptive nor expressive language deficits are included in these diagnostic criteria, but many individuals diagnosed with ASD exhibit difficulties in these areas, particularly those individuals whose autism is within the moderate to severe range. Identity-first language is used throughout this chapter, in deference to self-advocates within the Autistic community.

Approximately 30% of Autistic individuals will remain minimally speaking (Tager-Flusberg & Kasari, 2013). Among those who do develop some spoken language, patterns observed include a limited expressive vocabulary with an overrepresentation of nouns, delayed or disordered syntax, and scripted speech (Shane et al., 2014; Tager-Flusberg et al., 2005). Many individuals with moderate to severe ASD also demonstrate difficulties understanding spoken language (Muller & Brady, 2016; Weismer et al., 2010; Shane et al., 2014). The receptive language skills among children with moderate to severe ASD are often characterized by a relative strength comprehending nouns in both spoken and visual form (Kover & Weismer, 2014; Hudry et al., 2010), as well as poor comprehension of abstract and relational language components (e.g., prepositions and verbs) (Horwitz et al., 2014; Swensen et al., 2007). Therefore, when considering intervention strategies for children with moderate to severe ASD, it is crucial to target not only expressive communication, but also receptive language skills.

By the time Autistic children enter kindergarten, approximately 75% will use some spoken language (i.e., at least five spoken words a day) and about 50% will use phrase-based sentences (Anderson et al., 2007). Therefore, the majority of preschool-aged children with ASD are considered preverbal,

DOI: 10.4324/9781003106739-6

meaning they will eventually use at least some spoken language (Tager-Flusberg & Kasari, 2013). Nevertheless, it remains difficult to accurately identify those children who will remain nonspeaking or minimally speaking. It is also difficult to predict if the spoken language preverbal children acquire will meet the full range of their communicative needs (e.g., requesting, commenting, giving directives, etc.).

Considering that many Autistic individuals demonstrate a strength in visual processing (Ashwin et al., 2009; Thaut, 1987), alternative and augmentative communication (AAC) strategies can serve as a compensatory strategy for expressive and receptive language deficits. Given the variability in language skills and the difficulty predicting language outcomes, it is important that the AAC strategies introduced support those children who will eventually acquire spoken language and those who will not.

The Visual Immersion System

The Visual Immersion System™ (VIS™) is a visually based assessment and treatment approach that integrates a variety of AAC strategies to support the comprehension of spoken language, the use of symbolic communication expressively, and the organization of tasks among Autistic individuals and those with other developmental disabilities (Shane et al., 2014). The VIS™ follows a developmental approach based on four guiding principles: (1) Autistic individuals demonstrate increased comprehension when spoken language is supplemented with a symbol-rich environment (Quill, 1997; Mesibov et al., 1994); (2) AAC strategies should promote multiple communicative functions (Prizant & Wetherby, 2005); (3) a developmental perspective should be used to identify appropriate tools within a child's zone of proximal development (as outlined in Table 6.1); and (4) visual supports should be immersive and integrated into other treatment approaches.

To create a comprehensive, visual communication system that supplements speech, the VIS™ uses visual supports delivered through high-tech, mid-tech, and low-tech AAC tools (Shane et al., 2014). The goal of the VIS™ is not to replace the spoken language of the learner or the communication partner, but to supplement it. The VIS™ distinguishes between three modes of visual supports (see Shane & Weiss-Kapp, 2008):

1. *Visual Expressive Mode (VEM):* Visual supports used for the purpose of expressive communication (e.g., choice board).
2. *Visual Instructional Mode (VIM):* Visual supports used for comprehension, as an alternative to, or in conjunction with, auditory input (e.g., photographs paired with spoken language).
3. *Visual Organizational Mode (VOM):* Visual supports to aid executive functioning by representing the organization or an activity, routine, script, or schedule (e.g., visual schedule).

Table 6.1 The Visual Immersion System™ Developmental Stages in Symbolic Communication Skills

Phase	Learner Phase	Description
I	Presymbolic communicator	Learner is pre-intentional and communication partners attribute meaning to nonverbal behaviours. Learner is beginning to understand communicative intents have an impact on their immediate environment
II	Concrete symbolic communicator	Learner is demonstrating emerging symbolic communication skills by using a concrete reference (e.g., 3D object or symbol) intentionally to communicate
III	Context-based symbolic communicator	Learner comprehends use of photograph representations and visual scene displays that accurately depict their environment
IV	Emerging abstract symbolic communicator	Learner is beginning to combine abstract symbols with real photographs to increase mean length of utterance
V	Abstract symbolic communicator	Learner comprehends use of abstract symbols, no longer requires context-based visual supports, and is using pre-elementary grid-based visual supports for communication
VI	Generative symbolic communicator	Learner has a strong comprehension of abstract symbol formats within a grid-based system and creates novel phrases of increasing length and complexity

When implemented with preschool- to early elementary-aged Autistic children, the VIS™ has three possible outcomes: (1) visual supports are faded out following the development of spoken language, (2) visual supports continue to supplement receptive and expressive language, or (3) AAC becomes the individual's primary form of communication.

A Dynamic Assessment Approach

The VIS™ framework adopts a dynamic assessment approach to identify appropriate AAC methods for children diagnosed with moderate to severe ASD (Yu et al., 2017; Shane et al., 2014), identifying goals within a child's zone of proximal development by informally assessing the child's current speech and language skills and then providing scaffolding during clinician-led activities and comparing changes in performance with these modifications (Haywood, 2007; Poehner & Lantolf, 2010; Kasari et al., 2013). The process for identifying appropriate AAC tools typically incorporates caregiver report, direct observation of an individual's unaided communication, informal assessment of the individual's symbolic understanding, and informal language assessments with and without AAC supports (Yu et al., 2017). A dynamic assessment approach is especially important for Autistic children who are minimally speaking, as standardized tests rarely capture the language abilities of these children accurately due to challenges in behavior and engagement, as well as difficulty establishing rapport (Kasari et al., 2013). Additionally, creating meaningful treatment plans using information from standardized assessments alone can be challenging (Brady & Thiemann-Bourque, 2014). The recommendations for appropriate AAC tools determined during a dynamic assessment may allow for easier creation of goals given the child's predicted trajectory on a developmental framework (Yu et al., 2017).

This case report describes a dynamic assessment approach to identify appropriate AAC tools within the VIS™ for a preschool-aged Autistic child. It highlights the importance of identifying symbols that are understood by the learner when introducing AAC strategies. It also demonstrates the importance of targeting not only expressive language skills, but also receptive language skills during language intervention for Autistic children.

Presenting Concerns

When first seen, Jack was aged four years, three months and had a diagnosis of ASD. He was born without complications following a healthy, full-term pregnancy. A frenectomy was performed when Jack was two years old. No other hospitalizations or surgeries were reported. Jack's mother reported that his motor development was within normal limits, though his communication skills were delayed after initial milestones were met (e.g., vocal play and babbling). Medical records indicated no concerns regarding his hearing, vision, nutrition, or sleep. Jack did not take medications, and had no history of seizure activity, or of trauma. There was no family history of ASD. Jack's father had a diagnosis of attention deficit hyperactivity disorder (ADHD), and Jack's paternal uncle was reported to have a language delay as a child.

Jack was diagnosed with ASD at age two years, 11 months following an evaluation by a neurologist. His diagnosis was based, in part, on parent report and direct observation of decreased social-emotional reciprocity, nonverbal communication deficits, a lack of age-appropriate play, significant repetitive behaviors, restricted interests, and sensory seeking behaviors.

Jack lived at home with his parents and younger sister. He attended public school in a substantially separate classroom with eight other students, one teacher, and two paraprofessionals. At school, Jack received individual speech and language therapy for 30 minutes twice a week and occupational therapy for 30 minutes a week. The speech and language goals described in his Individualized Education Plan (IEP) addressed articulation and using a total communication approach to make requests. Occupational therapy goals addressed improvement of visual-motor skills with minimal physical assistance and using self-calming techniques to improve his sensory modulation (e.g., manipulating a tactile support). Jack also received 20 hours of home-based applied behavioral analysis (ABA) therapy. His primary ABA goals included (1) using the manual sign for "All done," (2) matching photographs to objects, and (3) utilizing the Picture Exchange Communication System (PECS) and manual signs to make requests.

Jack's parents identified communication as their biggest area of concern for Jack. Their primary goal was for Jack to clearly communicate his needs and wants to a variety of communication partners. Jack's board-certified behavior analyst (BCBA) introduced the Picture Exchange Communication System (PECS) when Jack was aged three. Over the course of a year, he mastered Phase II of PECS, meaning he initiated symbol exchanges independently using a variety of symbols presented one at a time (Bondy & Frost, 1994). Parents reported that he was currently at Phase III: Simultaneous Discrimination of Pictures of PECS, which requires the learner to discriminate between two or more symbols to request a desired object (Bondy & Frost, 1994).

His mother expressed concerns about a potential diagnosis of a sensory processing disorder and has discussed this issue with his school occupational therapist. Jack often demonstrated sensory seeking behaviors, including mouthing objects and spinning and he was reported to benefit from use of a weighted blanket to help him attend to a task. Without access to these supports, or the ability to receive additional sensory stimuli, he became dysregulated and could not actively engage in activities. Jack had previously engaged in self-injurious behaviors (i.e., head banging, seemingly to protest transitions to nonpreferred activities). His mother requested additional guidance related to sensory supports that could be integrated throughout their home, as she was worried that he might engage in self-injurious behaviors in the future.

Clinical Findings

Jack participated in an AAC evaluation in an outpatient hospital setting. His mother and father were present throughout and served as informants. The goal was to identify AAC tools that would support the development of Jack's receptive and expressive language skills. Formal standardized tests were not utilized due to the aforementioned difficulties in obtaining valid results among individuals diagnosed with moderate to severe ASD.

Based on parent interview and direct observation, Jack's existing communication skills were applied to the *Visual Immersion System® Communicative Operations Framework*, as outlined in Table 6.2.

This framework was developed to identify the modes of communication an individual uses to meet seven operations, which include six pragmatic functions and one executive-function skill (Shane et al., 2014).

1. *Protesting:* Jack's parents reported that he used physical communication (e.g., pushed items away), shook his head "no," the manual sign for "All Done," and a vocal approximation for "No" to protest. Jack was observed to push away materials to protest during his assessment.
2. *Making Requests:* Jack was reported to use physical communication (e.g., lead his communication partner by the hand to a desired object), gestures (e.g., point to a snack to request it), PECS (e.g., hand his communication partner a symbol to request goldfish crackers), and vocalizations (i.e., vowel

Table 6.2 Visual Immersion System® Communicative Operations Framework

Pragmatic Function	Definition	Example Modalities
Protesting	Communication to indicate the rejection of an object, activity, or person, or the cessation of an activity.	• Behaviors (e.g., running away) • Physical communication (e.g., pushing items away) • Gestures (e.g., shaking head "no") • Vocalizations • Speech (e.g., "No!") • Manual Signs (e.g., "All done") • Low-tech AAC strategies (e.g., picture symbol) • Mid-tech AAC device (e.g., "No" on GoTalk 9+) • Speech-generating device(s)
Requesting (known as a "mand" in applied behavioral analysis parlance)	Communication to obtain something (e.g., object, activity, food, etc.), gain attention or affection, the continuation of something, and/or assistance.	• Behaviors (e.g., sitting at the kitchen table to request food) • Physical communication (e.g., pulls communication partner to the door to request going outside) • Eye gaze (e.g., looking at a desired object) • Gestures (e.g., points to desired object) • Vocalizations • Speech • Manual signs (e.g., "more") • Low-tech AAC strategies (e.g., picture symbol for preferred snack) • Mid-tech AAC device • Speech-generating device(s)
Declarations and Commenting (known as a "tact" in applied behavioral analysis parlance)	Communication to call a communication partner's attention to something, comment on objects or the environment, and/or social comments.	• Physical communication (e.g., bringing an object to their communication partner to show them) • Gestures (e.g., points to show their communication partner something, like a plane in the sky) • Vocalizations • Speech • Manual signs (e.g., signing "ball" to label the toy they are playing with)

(Continued)

Table 6.2 (Continued)

Pragmatic Function	Definition	Example Modalities
Giving Directives	Communication with the intent of directing a communication partner.	• Low-tech AAC strategies (e.g., picture symbol to label an object in their environment) • Mid-tech AAC device (e.g., GoTalk 9+ with the social comment, "Cool!") • Speech-generating device(s) (e.g., "It + is + snowing") • Physical communication (e.g., putting their communication partner's hand on their stomach to give the directive, "Tickle me") • Gestures • Vocalizations • Speech • Manual signs (e.g., signing "open" to direct someone to open an item) • Low-tech AAC strategies (e.g., picture symbol of "push" to direct their communication partner to push them while on the swing) • Mid-tech AAC device • Speech-generating device(s) (e.g., "Come" on the homepage of TouchChat WordPower 42)
Asking Questions	Communication to gain information from a communication partner.	• Physical communication (e.g., bringing an object to an adult to indicate 'What is this?') • Gestures (e.g., raising hands to indicate 'why') • Vocalizations/speech approximations with a rising intonation • Speech (e.g., "Where's dad?") • Manual signs • Low-tech AAC strategies (e.g., using a topic display) • Mid-tech AAC device • Speech-generating device(s) (e.g., "Where are we going?")
Answering Questions	Communication in response to a question posed by a communication partner.	• Physical communication (e.g., pretending to sleep when asked, "What's the baby doing?") • Gestures (e.g., pointing to the ball when asked, "Where's the ball?") • Vocalizations/speech approximations • Speech (e.g., He is running," in response to someone asking, "What is the boy doing?) • Manual signs • Low-tech AAC strategies • Mid-tech AAC device • Speech-generating device(s)

Social Pragmatics	Communication to facilitate social exchanges to include greetings and partings, acknowledging what their communication partner says, demonstrating joint attention, following rules for conversation (e.g., turn-taking), observational learning skills, etc.	• Gestures (e.g., waving, tapping someone on the shoulder to gain attention) • Vocalizations • Speech • Manual signs (e.g., "Thank you") • Low-tech AAC strategies (e.g., conversation maps) • Mid-tech AAC device • Speech-generating device(s)
Following Directives	Comprehension and completion of a directive given by a communication partner (e.g., familiar one-step directives, related two-step directives, etc.).	• Gestures (e.g., saying "Pick up the book" while pointing to the book) • Visuals (e.g., playing a video model of someone washing their hands while saying "wash your hands") • Augmented input (e.g., "put + in" on a speech-generating device)
Transitioning	The process of moving from one activity or environment to another.	• Visual schedules • Timer • Countdown board • First/then displays (e.g., "First clean up, then iPad")

sounds) to make requests. During his assessment, Jack was observed to use physical communication to make a request (e.g., brought his mother to the door, then placed her hand on the doorknob to request leaving).

3. ***Following and Giving Directions:*** According to his parents, Jack followed routine-based, one-step directives (e.g., "Put your shoes on"). He was observed to give directives using physical communication (e.g., placed his mother's hand on his stomach to direct her to tickle him).

4. ***Commenting and Labeling:*** Jack's parents reported that he did not yet use symbolic communication to comment or label.

5. ***Asking and Answering Questions:*** Jack answered forced-choice questions when two food choices were held up by his communication partner (e.g., reached towards his choice when asked, "Do you want chips or goldfish?"). His parents reported that he did not yet ask questions.

6. ***Transitioning:*** Jack's parents noted that he had difficulty transitioning between environments and activities, especially when transitioning to something nonpreferred.

7. ***Social Pragmatics:*** Jack greeted others following an adult model. Jack reportedly participated in parallel play with his younger sister.

Diagnostic Assessment

Assessed Level of Symbolic Representation

The most common symbol types used to communicate are speech, manual signs or gestures, graphic symbols, orthography, and videos (Beukelman & Mirenda, 2013). Symbolic communication is dependent on an individual making associations between symbols and their referents. These associations are learned through exposure and/or direct instruction (Robinson & Griffith, 1979).

Aided symbols require some kind of device or materials that are external to the human body (Lloyd & Fuller, 1986). Aided symbols can be two-dimensional (2-D; e.g., line drawings) or three-dimensional (3-D; e.g., objects). Iconicity refers to the ease with which symbols can be recognized (Lloyd & Fuller, 1990). In general, 3-D object proxies are regarded as the most iconic symbol form, followed by photographs accurately depicting an environment, photographs with the background context removed, color line drawings, and black-and-white line drawings (e.g., picture communication symbols), abstract line drawings (e.g., lexigrams), and traditional orthography, as shown in Figure 6.1 (Lloyd et al., 1997; Shane et al., 2014).

Typically developing children recognize objects in photographs between 9 and 18 months old and understand the use of photographs as symbols by 19 months old (Murphy, 1978; DeRoche et al., 1998; Preissler & Carey, 2004; Yonas et al., 2005). Preliminary research on selecting graphic symbols for Autistic children suggests that iconic rather than opaque symbols should be considered when introducing symbols for the purpose of requesting (Kozleski, 1991; Schlosser & Sigafoos, 2009). To determine Jack's developmental level of

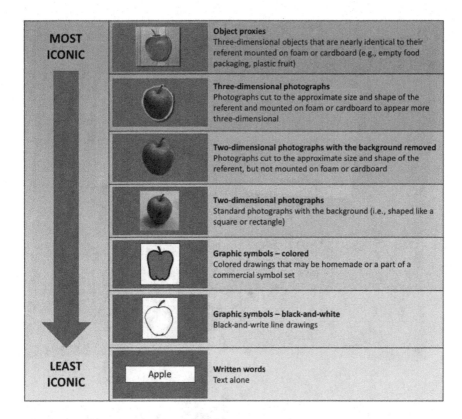

Figure 6.1 Iconicity continuum in symbolic communication

symbolic understanding, he was presented with three different symbol levels on the continuum, beginning with the most iconic.

1. **Objects:** Jack was presented with a sorting and matching task that required him to differentiate between two 3-D objects (e.g., toy whales and turtles) and place them into corresponding bins. Jack independently sorted 10/10 objects, indicating an understanding of categorical distinction with physical objects.
2. **Photographs with background present:** Jack was next presented with a field of two 3- × 3-inch photographs representing a preferred object (e.g., bubbles container) and a nonpreferred object (e.g., sock) to assess his symbolic understanding of 2-D photographs and their intended 3-D referent. The laminated photographs were attached horizontally with Velcro to an 8- × 11-inch choice board, as shown in Figure 6.2.

    When shown the 3-D bubbles container, Jack was instructed to point to or remove the matching photograph to request bubbles. If he pointed to the photograph of a nonpreferred item, he was given a 3-D sock.

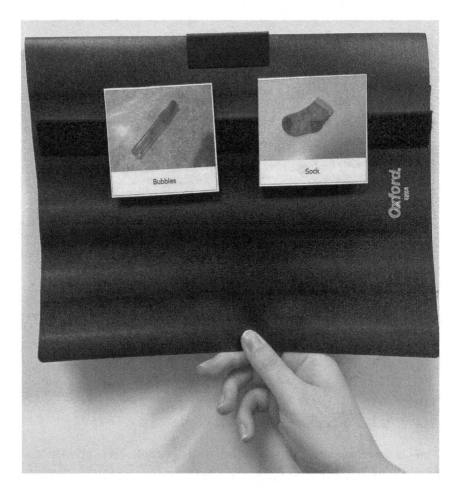

Figure 6.2 Example of laminated photographs on a choice board

Initially, Jack did not attend to the photographs and attempted to obtain the physical bubbles container from the clinician. When provided with direct modeling, Jack matched the bubbles photograph to the bubble container on two occasions; however, he also selected the photograph of the nonpreferred item on the following opportunity. To assess communication intentionality, this activity was continued by changing the position of the photographs position (i.e., left vs. right) and orientation (i.e., horizontally vs. vertically). Overall, Jack selected the bubbles photograph in 7/10 opportunities, indicating emerging understanding of 2-D photograph to 3-D object relationships.

3. **Graphic symbols:** Jack had previously been exposed to PECS with graphic symbols (i.e., color line drawings). To assess Jack's symbolic understanding

of 2-D graphic symbols to objects, he was presented with the same matching task, but now with a field of two 3 x 3-inch graphic symbols representing the preferred and nonpreferred objects. Jack consistently selected the graphic symbol placed on the right, regardless of whether this was his preferred option. This suggested that Jack did not yet associate graphic symbols with their 3-D referent.

AAC Identified Tools to Support Receptive and Expressive Language Skills

Once Jack's level of symbolic representation was identified, the following VIS™ tools were used during test and retest informal language assessments.

- **Noun Element Cues:** Noun element cues are 2-D photographs of object representations that support comprehension of spoken directives and questions (e.g., the directive, "Give me the ball" paired with a photograph of the ball). Jack was presented with noun element cues to assess his ability to follow spoken directives with visual supports. Five figurines were arranged on the table. With a spoken directive paired with a gesture (e.g., "Give me the dog" and a hand reaching out), Jack did not respond across three opportunities. When the spoken directives were paired with a noun element cue on an iPad and a gesture ("Give me the dog" + picture of dog + a hand reaching out), Jack independently found the correct figurine in a field of five and presented it to the clinician in four of five trials.
- **Dynamic Scene Cues:** Dynamic scene cues are full-motion video clips depicting underlying relevant concepts and their relationships that are paired with spoken directives to support language comprehension and imitation (Schlosser et al., 2013). Jack was presented with several figurines and given one-step spoken directives (e.g., "Put the bear in the plane"). Directives that were not completed were repeated using spoken language alone up to three times. Jack was not observed to follow the four one-step directives. To support Jack's ability to complete directives, dynamic scene cues were presented to Jack in conjunction with spoken directives (e.g., the spoken directive, "Put the bear in the plane" paired with a video of the bear being put in the plane). Jack readily attended to the iPad and independently completed four of the six (~66%) one-step directives given.
- **Grid Displays:** Grid displays arrange multiple symbols (e.g., photographs or graphic symbols) into rows and columns. Individual symbols in grid display often represent nouns, verbs, attributes, spatial and temporal concepts, and questions in isolation. This allows the user to make choices or combine symbols into multiword phrases or sentences. Jack was presented with a four-location grid display within the *GoTalk NOW* application on an iPad for the purpose of requesting. The symbols in the grid consisted of photographs of objects with no contextual background to focus attention on the object by eliminating "noise." Jack required hand-over-hand support to select his desired item (e.g., bubbles). Without assistance, he did not visually scan options and appeared to make selections randomly.

- ***Visual Scene Displays:*** Visual scene displays (VSDs) are photographs that depict environments, objects, activities, actions and/or people, and that allow users to touch "hot spots" on the photograph to speak messages relating to the scene (Blackstone, 2005). They provide increased context compared to a grid display and can provide opportunity for errorless learning. Jack was presented with VSDs within the *GoTalk NOW* application on an iPad. Using an isolated index finger, Jack initially depressed targets without waiting for the screen to output a verbal message. Built-in application access settings were modified, including programming a debounce period (i.e., disabling on-screen items for 0.5 seconds following an item selection) to reduce repetitive tapping behaviors and accidental item selection. Additionally, iOS Guided Access (https://support.apple.com/en-us/HT202612) was enabled to prevent Jack from performing on-screen gestures and using physical iPad buttons that would navigate out of the application.

  - ***Bubbles (1 hotspot):*** When presented with a bubbles VSD, Jack activated the display to request "blow bubbles," initially with gestural and spoken cues, fading to the point of independence in four opportunities.
  - ***Puzzle (8 hot spots):*** When presented with a VSD of a puzzle, Jack was directed to label and/or request animal pieces using the hotspots. Following initial gestural and spoken modeling, Jack selected five out of eight (62.5%) hotspots on the display to label the animal puzzle pieces.

- ***The Boston Children's Hospital Teaching Imitation Program:*** To assess Jack's imitation skills, he was presented with the *Boston Children's Teaching Imitation Program*, which consists of videos of agents performing simple body actions or actions containing one or more objects. Jack was shown videos of basic body actions and actions containing one or more objects and encouraged to imitate the on-screen model when told, "Do this." Jack visually attended to the screen without prompting and independently imitated the following actions: clapping, hands on head, jumping, waving, and shaking hands. When presented with an agent performing an action relating one or more objects, Jack independently imitated the following actions: place a towel on your head, crumple a piece of paper and throw it across the room, and place a cup upside down.

Therapeutic Intervention

Assessment of Jack's level of symbolic understanding indicated he was a context-based symbolic communicator, meaning that photograph representations accurately depicting his immediate environment were within his zone of proximal development to support symbolic communication. Based on the *Visual Immersion System® Communicative Operations Framework* (Shane et al., 2014), Jack's therapeutic intervention needed to focus on increasing his consistency using symbolic communication to make requests, label objects in his environment, and imitate one-step play actions. The tools best suited to these goals included noun elements, dynamic scene cues, and visual scene displays.

The VIS™ is not intended to replace other treatment models used for Autistic individuals, but rather to complement and be integrated into these treatment approaches. It is most effective when an individual's environment becomes visually immersive, offering frequent and varied visual supports. Therefore, successful implementation of the VIS™ requires collaboration among parents, classroom teachers, speech-language pathologists, ABA therapists, and occupational therapists. Ideally, the visual tools created for Jack would be utilized across settings and throughout all structured activities to promote generalization.

The Visual Instructional Mode (VIM) tools identified to support Jack's receptive language skills were noun elements, dynamic scene cues, and visual scene displays. Noun elements (i.e., 2-D photographs of objects) were recommended to support the development of Jack's receptive vocabulary and his comprehension of spoken labels for everyday people, places, and objects by providing a clear referent onto which to map spoken labels. The following goal was incorporated into Jack's IEP: "Given a spoken directive to find a specific object paired with a visual support (i.e., photograph of common noun), Jack will independently follow the directive in 4 out of 5 measurable opportunities."

Based on Jack's imitation of videos during his assessment, dynamic scene cues were recommended to support directive following and the acquisition of new play skills and activities of daily living. Full-motion videos of dynamic scene cues can depict abstract, relational concepts (e.g., verbs, prepositions) as a form of augmented input during spoken directives (Allen et al., 2017; Shane, 2006). Personalized short videos of a model acting on one or two objects (e.g., make the toy dinosaur jump) can be presented on an electronic device (i.e., phone, tablet, computer). This should first be practiced during structured therapy sessions prior to generalizing to daily routines (e.g., put the bowl in the sink). The following goal was incorporated into Jack's IEP: "Following a dynamic scene cue and spoken directive, Jack will imitate at least 3 pretend play skills/language concepts (e.g., push the car, feed the doll) in 4 out of 5 measurable opportunities."

The primary Visual Expressive Mode (VEM) tool identified for Jack was VSDs programmed with speech output within an application capable of creating visual scene displays. Prior to Jack's evaluation, one of his ABA goals was to use PECS to make requests. During Phase I and Phase II of PECS, Jack used symbols to request highly preferred objects (e.g., Goldfish crackers, bubbles, etc.) by handing his communication partner the single symbol made available to him. While this may demonstrate that Jack recognized several graphic symbols, it is possible he was not visually attending to the symbols available to him. Jack's IEP goals for communication included making requests using a total communication approach. Both Jack's ABA goal and communication goal included making requests, which is an appropriate target considering his reliance on physical communication for making requests. Rather than using

PCS symbols, it was recommended that Jack's intervention integrate VSDs with speech output. The following goal was included in an addendum to Jack's IEP: "Using a visual scene display, Jack will select 5 pre-programmed words for the purposes of requesting or labeling with minimal support (e.g., spoken or gestural cue) in 4 out of 5 measurable opportunities across six consecutive sessions."

Follow-up and Outcomes

Jack returned for a speech-language evaluation six months later (see Timeline, Figure 6.3). At this time, Jack's parents noted that he frequently used visual scene displays for making requests for food, toys, and places, as well as labeling objects in his environment when prompted. They also reported an increase in his spoken production (i.e., speech approximations for approximately 10 words), although these approximations were only understood by familiar communication partners. Parents also reported improvements in Jack's play skills. For example, he now showed interest in his sister's play (i.e., would observe her play and would imitate certain actions, particularly gross motor actions). Finally, Jack's parents reported that his levels of frustration had been reduced since the introduction of the AAC tools. Despite these positive outcomes, they also expressed concern that Jack was only requesting, and they hoped that he would begin initiating social interactions with his peers and making comments spontaneously. They were encouraged by his increased spoken output and wanted to know how they could support his speech development. They reported the most difficult component of implementing the AAC tools was the spontaneous creation of materials that was sometimes required. Initially, they found the creation of visual scene displays difficult, and they required additional programming guidance from Jack's school speech-language pathologist.

During Jack's return speech-language evaluation, gains were observed in the frequency and effectiveness of symbolic requests, size of receptive vocabulary for nouns, and the use of symbolic communication to request and label objects in his environment when prompted. His evaluation indicated he was now an emerging abstract symbolic communicator. While this reflected an improvement in Jack's level of symbolic understanding, it remained important that he continued to use iconic symbols. Jack could now transition from a visual scene display layout to individual language elements in a grid display, as he no longer relied on the context of a specific environment to identify objects in photographs.

Following his initial evaluation, Jack had been referred to an occupational therapist specializing in sensory processing disorders to discuss the development of partner-based and independently initiated sensory strategies that could be utilized throughout Jack's primary environments. To create a plan that would fit his needs, he required an assessment to determine the specific sensory feedback he was seeking or avoiding (e.g., proprioceptive, vestibular,

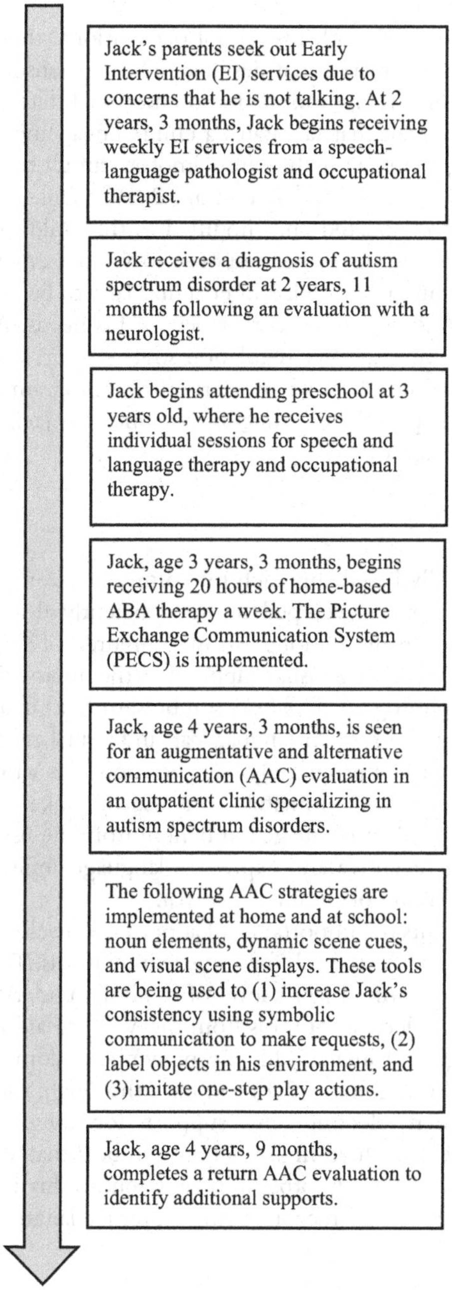

Jack's parents seek out Early Intervention (EI) services due to concerns that he is not talking. At 2 years, 3 months, Jack begins receiving weekly EI services from a speech-language pathologist and occupational therapist.

Jack receives a diagnosis of autism spectrum disorder at 2 years, 11 months following an evaluation with a neurologist.

Jack begins attending preschool at 3 years old, where he receives individual sessions for speech and language therapy and occupational therapy.

Jack, age 3 years, 3 months, begins receiving 20 hours of home-based ABA therapy a week. The Picture Exchange Communication System (PECS) is implemented.

Jack, age 4 years, 3 months, is seen for an augmentative and alternative communication (AAC) evaluation in an outpatient clinic specializing in autism spectrum disorders.

The following AAC strategies are implemented at home and at school: noun elements, dynamic scene cues, and visual scene displays. These tools are being used to (1) increase Jack's consistency using symbolic communication to make requests, (2) label objects in his environment, and (3) imitate one-step play actions.

Jack, age 4 years, 9 months, completes a return AAC evaluation to identify additional supports.

Figure 6.3 Timeline of intervention

tactile) and how his needs could be met while balancing his participation in daily activities.

Through collaboration with his school occupational therapist and his family, a sensory diet was created that designated which sensory activities best fit Jack's needs based on his environment and emotional state. A sensory diet is a customized sensory plan that facilitates a child's engagement in daily occupations by providing them with the sensorimotor stimuli they need to actively attend and remain regulated (Pinagle et al., 2019). This intervention is a living document that is updated and modified as the child grows and needs to be reevaluated based on his or her response to various environmental stimuli. Having multiple strategies was vital in enabling Jack to be an active participant in choosing activities and supports that best fit his needs. Additionally, visual scene displays depicting sensory regulation strategies were created. For example, a photograph of his school's sensory room was programmed with hot spots for "swing," "quiet space," and "squeezes" to increase Jack's independence in requesting sensory supports.

Conclusion

The VIS™ is a visually based approach for communication and language intervention and assessment, developed to be sufficiently flexible to address the variety in language profiles among Autistic children. The foundation of the VIS™ involves incorporating visual supports at the appropriate symbolic level for a learner (e.g., photographs, picture symbols, or text) in an immersive manner to complement the spoken language an individual receives (Shane et al., 2014). Therefore, with appropriately selected tools, the VIS™ can serve young Autistic children who will ultimately gain use of spoken language, children who will use some spoken language but benefit from the use of AAC strategies to strengthen their receptive and expressive language abilities, and those who will remain nonspeaking or minimally verbal.

Jack's case highlights the importance of adopting a developmental perspective to identify appropriate AAC tools for Autistic individuals. The VIS™ assessment process accurately identified Jack's level of symbolic understanding, which, in turn, informed the selection of tools from the VIS™ to aid his comprehension of spoken language and increase his use of symbolic communication expressively. Jack's case also highlights the need for a thorough, individualized assessment approach when selecting AAC supports for individuals with complex communication needs. Once highly iconic symbols that were meaningful to Jack were introduced (i.e., photographs representing his immediate environment), he made gains in his receptive and expressive language skills.

References

Allen, A. A., Schlosser, R. W., Brock, K. L., & Shane, H. C. (2017). The effectiveness of aided augmented input techniques for persons with developmental disabilities: A systematic review. *Augmentative and Alternative Communication, 33,* 149–159. https://doi.org/10. 1080/07434618.2017.1338752

American Psychiatric Association. (2013). *The Diagnostic and statistical manual of mental disorders* (5th ed.). American Psychiatric Association.

Anderson, D., Lord, C., Risi, S., DiLavore, P., Shulman, C., Thurm, A., . . . Pickles, A. (2007). Patterns of growth in verbal abilities among children with autism spectrum disorder. *Journal of Consulting and Clinical Psychology, 75*(4), 594–604. https://psycnet.apa.org/ doi/10.1037/0022-006X.75.4.594

Ashwin, E., Ashwin, C., Rhydderch, D., Howells, J., & Baron-Cohen, S. (2009). Eagle-eyed visual acuity: An experimental investigation of enhanced perception in autism. *Biological Psychiatry, 65*(1), 17–21. https://doi.org/10.1016/j.biopsych.2008.06.012

Beukelman, D., & Mirenda, P. (2013). *Augmentative and alternative communication: Supporting children and adults with complex communication needs* (4th ed.). Brookes Publishing Co.

Blackstone, S. (2005). What are visual scene displays? *Augmentative Communication News, 16,* 2.

Bondy, A., & Frost, L. (1994). The picture exchange communication system. *Focus on Autistic Behavior, 9,* 1–19. https://doi.org/10.1177%2F108835769400900301

Brady & Thiemann-Bourque. (2014, November). *Outline for assessment and treatment of nonverbal or minimally verbal children with autism and other neurodevelopmental disabilities.* Seminar presented at the annual convention of the American Speech- Language-Hearing Association (ASHA).

DeRoche, J. S., Pierroutsakos, S. L., Uttal, D. H., Rosengren, K. S., & Gottlieb, A. (1998). Grasping the nature of pictures. *Psychological Science, 9,* 205–210. https://doi. org/10.1111/1467-9280.00039

Haywood, H., C. (2007). New models of ability are needed: New methods of assessment will be required. *Primate Perspectives on Behavior and Cognition,* 125–134.

Horwitz, L., McCarthy, J., Roth, M., & Marinellie, S. (2014). The effects of an animated exemplar/nonexemplar program to teach the relational concept *on* to children with autism spectrum disorders and developmental delays who require AAC. *Contemporary Issues in Communication Science and Disorders, 41,* 83–95. http://dx.doi.org/10.1044/ cicsd_41_s_83" \t "10.1044/cicsd_41_s_83

Hudry, K., Leadbitter, K., Temple, K., Slonims, V., McConachie, H., Aldred, C., & Charman, T. (2010). Preschoolers with autism show greater impairment in receptive compared with expressive language abilities. *International journal of Language & Communication Disorders, 45*(6), 681–690. https://doi.org/10.3109/13682820903461493

Kasari, C., Brady, N., Lord, C., & Tager-Flusberg, H. (2013). Assessing the minimally verbal school-aged child with autism spectrum disorder. *Autism Research, 6*(6), 479–493. https:// doi.org/10.1002/aur.1334

Kover, S., & Weismer, S. E. (2014). Lexical characteristics of expressive vocabulary in toddlers with autism spectrum disorder. *Journal of Speech, Language and Hearing Research, 57*(4), 1428–1441.

Kozleski, E. B. (1991). Visual symbol acquisition by students with autism. *Exceptionality, 2,* 173–194.

Lloyd, L., & Fuller, D. (1986). Toward an augmentative and alternative communication symbol taxonomy: A proposed superordinate classification. *Augmentative and Alternative Communication, 2*(4), 165–171. https://doi.org/10.1080/07434618612331273990

Lloyd, L., & Fuller, D. (1990). The role of iconicity in augmentative and alternative communication symbol learning. In W. Fraser (Ed.), *Key issues in mental retardation research* (pp. 295–306). Routledge.

Lloyd, L. L., Fuller, D. R., & Arvidson, H. (1997). *Augmentative and alternative communication: A handbook of principles and practices.* Allyn & Bacon Publishing Company.

Maenner, M. J., Shaw, K. A., Baio, J., Washington, A., Patrick, M., DiRienzo, M., et al. (2020). Prevalence of autism spectrum disorder among children aged 8 years – autism and developmental disabilities monitoring network, 11 sites, United States, 2016. *MMWR Surveillance Summaries, 69*(SS–4), 1–12. https://dx.doi.org/10.15585%2Fmmwr.ss6904a

Mesibov, G. B., Schopler, E., & Hearsey, K. (1994). Structured teaching. In E. Schopler & G. B. Mesibov (Eds.), *Behavioral issues in Autism* (pp. 195–207). Plenum Press.

Muller, K., & Brady, N. (2016). Assessing early receptive language skills in children with ASD. *Perspectives of the ASHA Special Interest Groups, 1*(1), 12–19. https://doi.org/10.1044/persp1.SIG1.1

Murphy, C. M. (1978). Pointing in the context of a shared activity. *Child Development, 49*, 371–380. https://doi.org/10.2307/1128700

Pinagle, V., Fletcher, T., & Candler, C. (2019). The effects of sensory diets on children's classroom behaviors. *Journal of Occupational Therapy, Schools, & Intervention, 12*(2), 225–238.

Plesa Skwerer, D., Jordan, S. E., Brukilacchio, B. H., & Tager-Flusberg, H. (2016). Comparing methods for assessing receptive language skills in minimally verbal children and adolescents with autism spectrum disorders. *Autism, 20*(5), 591–604. https://doi.org/10.1177/1362361315600146

Poehner, M. E., & Lantolf, J. P. (2010). Vygotsky's teaching-assessment dialectic and L2 education: Case for dynamic assessment. *Mind, Culture, and Activity, 17*(4), 312–330.

Preissler, M. A., & Carey, S. (2004). Do both pictures and words function as symbols for 18-month and 24-month-old children? *Journal of Cognition and Development, 5*, 185–212. https://doi.org/10.1207/s15327647jcd0502_2

Prizant, B. M., & Wetherby, A. M. (2005). Critical issues in enhancing communication abilities for persons with autism spectrum disorders. In F. R. Volkmar, R. Paul, A. Klin, & D. Cohen (Eds.), *Handbook of autism and pervasive developmental disorders: Assessment, interventions, and policy* (p. 925–945). John Wiley & Sons Inc. https://doi.org/10.1002/9780470939352.ch10

Quill, K. (1997). Instructional considerations for young children with autism: The rationale for visually cued instruction. *Journal of Autism and Developmental Disorders, 27*, 697–714.

Robinson, J. H., & Griffith, P. L. (1979). On the scientific status of iconicity. *Sign Language Studies, 25*, 297–315. www.jstor.org/stable/26203472

Schlosser, R., & Sigafoos, J. (2009). Selecting graphic symbols for an initial request lexicon: Integrative review. *Augmentative and Alternative Communication, 18*(2), 102–123.

Schlosser, R. W., Laubscher, E., Sorce, J., Koul, R., Flynn, S., Hotz, L., . . . Shane, H. (2013). Implementing directives that involve prepositions with children with autism: A comparison of spoken cues with two types of augmented input. *Augmentative and Alternative Communication, 29*, 132–145. https://doi.org/10.3109/07434618.2013.784928

Shane, H. C. (2006). Using visual scene displays to improve communication and communication instruction in persons with autism spectrum disorders. *Perspectives in Augmentative and Alternative Communication, 15*, 7–13. https://doi.org/10.1044/aac15.1.8

Shane, H., & Weiss-Kapp, S. (2008). *Visual Language in Autism.* Plural Publishing.

Shane, H. C., Laubscher, E., Schlosser, R. W., Fadie, H. L., Sorce, J. F., Abramson, J. S., . . . Corley, K. (2014). *Enhancing communication for individuals with autism.* Paul H. Brookes Publishing Co.

Swensen, L., Kelley, E., Fein, D., & Naigles, L. (2007). Processes of language acquisition in children with autism: Evidence from preferential looking. *Child Development, 78*(2), 542–557. https://doi.org/10.1111/j.1467-8624.2007.01022.x

Tager-Flusberg, H., & Kasari, C. (2013). Minimally verbal school-aged children with autism spectrum disorder: The neglected end of the spectrum. *Autism Research, 6*(6), 468–478. https://doi.org/10.1002/aur.1329

Tager-Flusberg, H., Paul, R., & Lord, C. E. (2005). Language and communication in autism. In F. Volkmar, R. Paul, A. Klin, D. J. Cohen (Eds.), *Handbook of autism and pervasive developmental disorder. 3* (Vol. 1). Wiley.

Thaut, M. H. (1987). Visual versus auditory (musical) stimulus preferences in autistic children: A pilot study. *Journal of Autism and Developmental Disorders, 17*(3), 425–432. https://doi.org/10.1007/BF01487071

Weismer, S. E., Lord, C., & Esler, A. (2010). Early language patterns of toddlers on the autism spectrum compared to toddlers with developmental delay. *Journal of Autism and Developmental Disorders, 40*(10), 1259–1273. http://doi.org/10.1007/s10803-010-0983-1

Yonas, A., Granrud, C. E., Chov, M. H., & Alexander, A. J. (2005). Picture perception in infants: Do 9-month-olds attempt to grasp objects depicted in photographs? *Infant Behavior and Development, 8*, 147–166. https://doi.org/10.1207/s15327078in0802_3

Yu, C., Shane, H., Schlosser, R., O'Brien, A., Allen, A., Abramson, J., . . . Flynn, S. (2017, November). *1733: Enhancing language in autism: Implementation of the visual immersion system™-developmental framework (VIS™-DF) in clinical practice.* Seminar presented at the annual convention of the American Speech-Language Hearing Association (ASHA).

7 Autism Spectrum Disorder, AAC, and the Feature-Matching Process

A Case Report

Molly B. Allen, Nicole Choe, Loren F. McMahon, Ralf W. Schlosser, Suzanne Flynn, Christina Yu and Howard C. Shane

Introduction

It is estimated that 20% to 30% of individuals with autism spectrum disorder (ASD) are nonspeaking or minimally verbal. Accordingly, these individuals produce no spoken output, use some speech approximations, or use a few single words and/or scripted phrases (Tager-Flusberg & Kasari, 2013). Their language profiles are diverse, with many evidencing difficulties comprehending spoken language and nonverbal cues. Additionally, there is often an absence of or reduced use of symbolic forms of expressive communication (e.g., overreliance on physical communication, limited gesture repertoire), and presence of challenging behaviors (Maljaars et al., 2011; McClintock et al., 2003; Tager-Flusberg et al., 2005).

One intervention approach often utilized with this population is AAC. Some are hesitant to use AAC due to concerns that AAC use could hinder speech development, but the use of AAC intervention strategies for individuals with developmental disabilities, including ASD, has been shown to have no negative impact on future speech development, and often promotes increased speech production (Millar et al., 2006; Schlosser & Wendt, 2008). In addition, the application of AAC can promote an increase in receptive vocabulary and language skills (Allen et al., 2017; Dada et al., 2020; Sennott et al., 2016). Both unaided and aided AAC modalities are beneficial for promoting language and communication development, as effective multimodal communication facilitates clear communication exchanges (Sigafoos & Drasgow, 2001). This chapter focuses on aided AAC, specifically a speech-generating device.

The process of prescribing an AAC device for individuals with complex communication needs requires a client-centered, data-driven approach to promote continued use of the device throughout the individual's lifespan. As many as 33% of AAC devices may be abandoned by users, with most being abandoned within three months of acquisition (Costello et al., 2017; Phillips & Zhao, 1993; Scherer & Galvin, 1994). Reasons for abandonment include lack of consideration of user/caregiver opinions and preferences, changing needs

DOI: 10.4324/9781003106739-7

of the user, and failure to match user needs with device features (Martin & McCormack, 1999; Phillips & Zhao, 1993). Whereas high-tech speech-generating technology was once only available in dedicated communication devices, ironically the widespread availability of communication apps on general-purpose, consumer-level devices (Shane et al., 2012), including tablets and computers, poses a new risk of abandonment, as easy access to a "quick fix" may lead providers to forgo a multidisciplinary, evidence-based approach to selecting an AAC system (Gosnell et al., 2011).

To ensure an appropriate match between an individual and an AAC device, it is essential to employ a systematic feature-matching process. As defined by Shane and Costello (1994), feature-matching entails identifying appropriate AAC techniques that will best support an individual's current and future communication needs based on their existing strengths. Domains to consider in feature matching include the patient's history, factors related to medical, sensory, motor, speech, language, educational, cognitive, and behavioral functioning, as well as financial, family/support, social/environmental, interpreted communications, and patient-centered factors (see Table 7.1). Relevant components of each are detailed in this chapter.

Table 7.1 Domains of Assessment for Feature Matching

Domain	Suggested Information to Collect/Consider
Client History	Previous medical, social, educational, vocational, environmental history; previous communication techniques and AAC interventions used
Medical	Medical diagnoses; seizure activity; current medications; reports/plan of care from other medical specialists (e.g., otolaryngology, orthopedics, feeding specialist, etc.)
Sensory	Vision concerns; hearing concerns; reports/plan of care from vision specialist, audiologist, etc.; sensory profile
Motor	Seating; positioning; gait control and analysis; strength of control of various limbs, and potential impact on interaction with communication supports
Speech	Presence/absence of speech; intelligibility; sound repertoire; stimulability; respiration; resonance; speech as primary vs. secondary means of communication
Language	Current levels of comprehension and expression; means of expression; purposes of communication; level of symbolic representation (e.g., physical object, 3-D photograph, 2-D photograph, line drawing, text); vocabulary size/contents; literacy skills; category knowledge
Educational	Type of classroom; curriculum focus; familiarity of school team and specialists with AAC; willingness of school team and specialists to implement AAC; literacy skills; learning style
Cognitive	Levels of representation; attention; memory; executive functioning; problem solving; arousal; intellectual disability; presence of learning disabilities; other comorbid conditions impacting cognition

(*Continued*)

Table 7.1 (Continued)

Domain	Suggested Information to Collect/Consider
Behavioral	Levels of frustration; antecedents and consequents; impact of other domains (e.g., medication, nutrition) on behavior; strategies used to address behavior (e.g., visual supports)
Financial	Sources of funding for high-tech device; responsibility for device programming, repair, and implementation
Family/Support	Acceptance of need for AAC; comfort with AAC and technology; advocacy skills; strengths and needs in relation to AAC; preferences; cultural considerations
Social/ Environmental	Acceptance of AAC across environments; types and consistency of social partners; access to peers; cultural considerations
Interpreted Communications	Behaviors, means of communication, etc., that are idiosyncratic or are only understood by familiar communication partners
Patient-Centered Factors	Patient/family concerns, goals, expectations, and preferences; patient personality and interests

Source: Adapted from Shane and Costello (1994) and Costello et al. (2017).

(For additional resources, see https://www.childrenshospital.org/programs/ augmentative-communication-program/downloads).

A multidisciplinary approach is key to ensuring that essential domains are appropriately addressed during the assessment process (Beukelman et al., 2008; Binger et al., 2012; Rose & McMahon, 2018). Speech, language, and literacy skills should be addressed by a speech-language pathologist (SLP). Mobility, tone, participation in activities of daily living, and seating/positioning should have inputs from an occupational therapist (OT). Additional realms, including cognition/attention, sensory skills, medical status, medications, nutrition, seizures, social support, neurological concerns, personal preferences and interests, etc., require input from all team members (e.g., client, family, SLP, OT, school team, primary care physician) to ensure all relevant information is considered when determining the appropriate AAC system (Costello et al., 2017; McMahon et al., 2019).

When considering varying communication systems and apps, it is important to analyze and compare the features of each system. Gosnell et al. (2011) grouped the fundamental features of communication systems that must be considered into 11 main categories (see Table 7.2). It is essential to identify the features that are critical for each individual to ensure that the selected communication system best matches their identified needs, and that it promotes functional communicative use and consistent implementation of the AAC system (Costello et al., 2017; Martin & McCormack, 1999; Shane & Costello, 1994).

Once an appropriate AAC system is identified, an evidence-based trial of at least 30 days is needed to ensure the system is an appropriate match for

Table 7.2 Fundamental Features of Communication Apps/Systems

Category	Description
Purpose of Use	Receptive, expressive, and/or organization
Output	Type of speech produced when using the communication system
Speech Settings	Volume, pitch, rate, and options for when the device speaks (e.g., speak after message selection or speak after each word)
Representation	Icon/symbol options, including orthography, graphic symbols, and/or photographs
Display	Layout (dynamic or static, scene-based displays or grid displays) and ability to change the size of symbols, font, color, and borders
Feedback Features	Input when an icon is presented (highlight, zoom, enlargement, auditory review) or when icon is selected (tactile, vibration)
Rate Enhancement	Strategies to increase the rate of communication output to increase efficiency, including word prediction, abbreviation expansion, recently used lists, grammar prediction, predictive linking
Access	How the user interacts with the device (e.g., direct selection, pointer, and/or scanning); customization options, including dwell time and keyguards
Motor Competencies	Motor abilities required to interact with the system, including pinching and/or swiping
Support	Resources that help users and care providers, including technical support and/or consultation
Miscellaneous	Options related to emailing, texting, phone calls, internet access, and/or web-based editing

Source: Adapted from Gosnell et al., 2011.

the individual. The trial process, usually led by an SLP, entails collecting data about the types and purposes of utterances constructed using this system across a variety of communication partners and settings (Shane & Costello, 1994). To promote communicative competence with a new AAC device, intervention goals for the trial should be established based on the four domains of communicative competence originally defined by Light (1989): (1) linguistic (i.e., having sufficient receptive and expressive language skills for both spoken language and the symbol "language" of the device); (2) operational (i.e., skills needed to physically access the device and operate device features); (3) social (i.e., following rules of communication interactions, utilizing various functions of communication); and (4) strategic (i.e., employing appropriate strategies to communicate a message clearly). These competencies provide a framework for evidence-based AAC intervention and help to support individuals in reaching their communicative potential (Light & McNaughton, 2014).

The following case report details how the feature-matching process was implemented to prescribe a high-tech AAC device for a young child with ASD. This included initial assessment using feature matching, device selection, evidence-based trial, outcomes, and follow-up measures.

Presenting Concerns

West is a 4-year, 3-month-old male with a medical history significant for ASD, Noonan syndrome, global developmental delays, pulmonary stenosis requiring multiple catheterizations and surgical repair, lymphedema, failure to thrive with gastrostomy tube in place, laryngo- and tracheomalacia, previous tracheostomy tube, and Noonan syndrome–associated juvenile myelomonocytic leukemia. While he does not present with seizure activity on an ambulatory electroencephalogram (EEG), episodes of staring and abnormal movements are regularly monitored for changes in presentation and/or frequency. He receives 80% of his nutrition orally and receives supplemental feedings via his G-tube. He wears corrective lenses to address exotropia and astigmatism. He has started to ambulate independently for short distances with supervision, but continues to require adult support (e.g., holding hand) most of the time.

West lives at home with his parents and three older brothers, two of whom also have an ASD diagnosis. He has in-home nursing support to address ongoing medical concerns (e.g., G-tube feedings, medication administration). He attends a substantially separate classroom four days a week for three hours a day at a local public elementary school. There, he has a 1:1 instructional aide who supports his participation in social, play, curriculum, and self-care activities. Through school, West receives weekly occupational therapy, speech and language therapy, physical therapy, and vision therapy, with consultative assistive technology services once a month. Outside of school, he receives private speech and language therapy (two or three 30-minute sessions each week), occupational therapy (one session every two weeks), feeding therapy (once a week), and applied behavior analysis (ABA) services (10 hours a week). West enjoys listening to music, playing with light-up toys, swinging, and watching TV shows and movies, especially those made by Disney.

West returned to an AAC specialist clinic with his family for his semiannual evaluation to assess current abilities and to obtain recommendations to further enhance his communication skills. Specifically, the family was interested in determining whether his current communication system still met his current and future needs. At the time of the evaluation, West was using a third-generation iPad Air™ running a communication app (i.e., GoTalk NOW™; www.attainmentcompany.com/gotalk-now) utilizing both grid- and visual scene displays as his primary means of communication. His vocabulary file contained grid displays only. These displays comprised a combination of choice-based pages and topic displays (i.e., vocabulary centered around one activity or area of interest). According to informal parent report and observation, West was able to use the device independently to request, but did not yet use the device to fulfill other communicative functions (e.g., protesting, directing others); additional means of communication included such behaviors as crying, throwing self on ground, and physical communication (e.g., pushing items away). Additionally, he required the device to be placed in iOS Guided Access during structured tasks to keep him from navigating out of his communication app to engage in leisure activities (e.g., watching videos). New pages had to be custom-made by his family members and other providers, as his communication app did not have a library of preset pages.

Clinical Findings

A comprehensive caregiver interview and informal assessment were completed prior to conducting the AAC portion of the evaluation, which consisted of dynamic assessment and observation. Relevant findings are outlined based on feature-matching domains.

Speech/Intelligibility

West did not produce any words or word approximations. His family had noted an increase in vocalizations/babbling over the last few months (e.g., "ma," and "ba") without apparent communicative intent.

Language Comprehension and Expression

West responded to his name, understood cause and effect, anticipated familiar routines, understood single words for familiar items and people, answered simple choice-based questions, followed routine one-step directions, and demonstrated emerging understanding of basic pre-academic concepts (e.g., colors, shapes). His family discussed a recent increase in his understanding of spoken language, as evidenced by his ability to follow spoken one-step directives.

Expressively, West was considered a multimodal communicator who used gestures, a limited repertoire of manual signs (e.g., MORE), physical communication (e.g., bringing communication partner to desired item), and an integrated AAC device (i.e., iPad Air™ used for both communication and leisure) running GoTalk NOW™.

His primary means of expression varied according to the purpose of his communication. He primarily protested using physical communication (e.g., pushing items away) or behavior (e.g., whining, throwing himself to the ground). He made single-word requests with his AAC device. He did not yet label items or ask questions. He answered choice-based "which" questions given objects or pictures by pointing at or grabbing his choice. West demonstrated an emerging ability to construct multiword directives using his AAC device during therapy sessions given clinician cueing. He required support from communication partners to say "hello" and "goodbye." He was interested in interacting with both peers and adults.

Although his family noted increases in West's receptive and expressive language skills, they also reported an increase in maladaptive behaviors (e.g., crying, throwing self on ground). Factors related to the maladaptive behaviors varied; they included lack of vocabulary in his AAC device, lack of an alternative means of expressing messages, and accidental selections made on his

AAC device because of physical access difficulties (e.g., inappropriate grasp). In these instances, communication breakdowns led to increased frustration, and he needed to work with his communication partners to clarify his message; this was often a painstaking and error-prone process, resulting in these breakdowns remaining unresolved most of the time.

Cognition

West benefited from a combination of real photographs and graphic symbols in his AAC device, with his strongest graphic symbol recognition being for iconic nouns (i.e., symbols for nouns that look identical or nearly identical to their physical referent). Given systematic, direct teaching using topic displays for motivating activities, he had started to learn and independently use graphic symbols for more abstract concepts (e.g., verbs, adjectives). His family reported that his attention to tasks varied widely depending on motivation and personal relevance of activities. His attention was also influenced by episodes of staring, related to possible seizure activity.

Sensory Function

West demonstrated functional vision with the support of corrective lenses and tolerated wearing glasses throughout the day. He was able to attend to materials and track items horizontally and vertically throughout the evaluation. He had no functional hearing concerns based on medical examination and family report, despite a history of repeated otitis media. Through previous activity analysis and participation in occupational therapy related to sensory integration and fine motor coordination, West presented with minimal tactile defensiveness while manipulating fine motor supports and integrating grasp patterns with novel tools during this evaluation.

Motor Function

West had diffuse hypotonia throughout his upper extremities resulting in decreased independent participation in activities of daily living (e.g., self-care, feeding). His axial hypotonia affected his mobility and gait, as well as his ability to participate unsupervised in dynamic standing activities. He had begun to ambulate independently for short distances, but required supervision due to an unsteady gait. He could ascend and descend stairs with bilateral hand holding with increased time. He benefited from the use of a manual commercial stroller for long distance mobility and transfers between environments.

West had a history of lower extremity lymphedema and received nightly manual lymph drainage with bilateral extremity wrapping and massage. He wore nighttime bilateral ankle foot orthoses to prevent calf contractures and support functional muscle range of motion from toe walking. Over the previous six months, West had an increased incidence of forward and backward falling with decreased righting reflex. His complex care team ran diagnostic testing including magnetic resonance imaging (MRI), computerized tomography (CT), and EEG to assess the cause of his falls. Potential causes included weakened trunk muscles paired with increased task demands when ambulating and performing dynamic activities, seizure activity, and vestibular dysfunction due to prolonged otitis media.

West is left-hand dominant. When interacting with physical tools and supports during this evaluation, he demonstrated functional motor performance skills in the context of iPad access as assessed using the *Occupational Therapy Practice Framework*: reaching, manipulation, gross motor coordination, digit isolation, stabilization, aligning, positioning, and calibration (American Occupational Therapy Association, 2014). He utilized an isolated left index finger as his primary access method when presented with interactive touch screen supports, as well as to physically gesture to preferred items. He occasionally used a raking, downward swipe on the screen when excited, requiring verbal prompts to return to an isolated digit. According to familial report and as observed during the assessment, his finger occasionally tended to slide when activating his device, resulting in accidental selections and visible frustration.

Educational

West's family reported that his school team had begun collaborating with his outside providers (e.g., private SLP) to address his AAC needs. The team continued to use his device (i.e., iPad Air™ with GoTalk NOW™) at school, with support from an assistive technology consultant. The team expressed willingness to implement any new AAC tools and strategies proposed during this evaluation given ongoing support from his outside AAC providers.

Family/Support

The primary goal of West's support system (e.g., family, providers) for this evaluation was to find an AAC system that would address his current communication needs and frustrations, as well as support language and communication growth over time. All parties were willing to learn and implement a new AAC system, if needed, to best suit his communication needs. His mother had served as the primary programmer for his current AAC device and was prepared to learn how to program a new device with continued support from his providers.

Patient-Centered Factors

West was an energetic boy who enjoyed physical play, listening to music, and watching a variety of children's TV shows, movies, and videos. He also demonstrated interest in engaging with both peers and adults. His current AAC system provided him with limited ability to engage with others beyond requesting. Therefore, finding an AAC system that would allow him to communicate with a variety of partners about his many interests was deemed essential to promoting continued "buy-in" from West. Additionally, teaching West how to use his device to repair communication breakdowns would be required to reduce frustration and encourage him to adopt a new AAC system as his own.

Diagnostic Assessment

West's ability to use his current AAC system (i.e., iPad Air™ running GoTalk NOW™) was assessed. He had a customized page set with a grid size of 16 items incorporating photographs and graphic symbols. West primarily used his AAC device to request. He generated novel two- to three-word/symbol combinations to give directives within structured activities if supported by his communication partner. He also independently navigated the page sets within his system using the left/right navigation buttons. During the evaluation, he accessed his device directly with an isolated left index finger; however, he made accidental item selections 30% of the time due to decreased coordination and intermittent use of a raking hand pattern (rather than isolated index finger selection). He became visibly frustrated upon accidental selection and was observed to make repetitive gestures on the iPad screen in an attempt to repair his message.

Principal shortcomings identified in West's current communication system included limited ability to communicate beyond requesting and a lack of a robust vocabulary system. To expand his current communication app to fit his current and future needs would require extensive programming and customization, as the app did not contain preprogrammed buttons or pages. As West's vocabulary and expressive language abilities were expected to continue expanding, he required a vocabulary that could grow with him. Therefore, it was determined that this app no longer met West's communication needs.

As outlined in Table 7.3, several necessary features of his future AAC system were identified based on his communication needs. Due to his growing receptive and expressive vocabulary, his future system needed to contain a robust vocabulary system, utilize a dynamic display, and contain customization options, including flexibility in symbol size, style (i.e., photographs and graphic symbols), font, and color. Because West's AAC device would be his primary communication tool, it also needed to include speech output. Due to his emerging ability to construct multiword utterances in his current communication system, it was determined that his future system should utilize predictive linking to encourage use of these combinations, as well as to promote rate acceleration. As a result of upper extremity physical motor limitations affecting direct access, his future system needed to allow for use of a keyguard and options to program a dwell time to reduce unintentional selections.

Table 7.3 Key Features Based on Assessment Outcomes

	Information Gathered During Assessment	*Key Requirements Identified Through Assessment*
Representation	Recognizes and can make choices using familiar photographs and graphic symbols	Photographs, graphic symbols Graphic symbols with text to support literacy development Ability to import photographs
Display Settings	Currently uses grid displays within grid-based communication app Is able to navigate dynamic displays with modeling	Dynamic display Ability to edit size/color/font of symbols and to hide buttons
Access/Motor	Direct selection with isolated index finger Frequent accidental item selections	Direct selection with isolated index finger Dwell Time: programmed at 0.3 seconds Keyguard: overlay with cut-outs to support item isolation; use resulted in decreased accidental selections
Support	Family requires support for training and resolving technical issues	Support/technical team
Purpose of Use	Primary communication tool Express a variety of communicative functions Expand expressive language Social engagement	Expressive tool Robust vocabulary system Predictive page linking for rate acceleration System that supports preprogrammed word and phrase-based message generation Synthesized voice output

Several communication systems and apps were considered based on the features that were identified to be critical for West's use (Table 7.4), including an iPad running a grid-based app with preset vocabulary libraries and predictive linking, and a dedicated device with a comparable communication app. West was first presented with a 20-button grid display within the iPad-based communication app. Given modeling, he navigated the dynamic display with a keyguard and generated novel two- to three-word/symbol utterances to request his preferred TV show. He was then presented with the 42-button grid display within the same communication app. His ability to accurately and intentionally access the buttons was reduced, even with a keyguard presented across multiple opportunities. Therefore, it was determined that the 20-button grid vocabulary file (Figure 7.1) would best fit West's communication and motor profile (Table 7.4). His use of this same vocabulary file within the dedicated device was comparable.

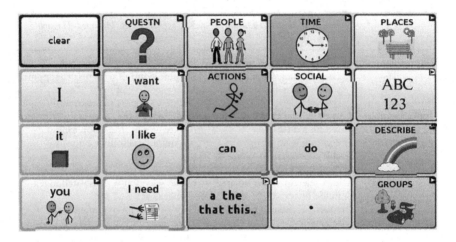

Figure 7.1 20-Button grid vocabulary file

Table 7.4 Summary of Key Clinical Findings and Diagnostic Assessment Results

Strengths	Areas of Challenge
Multimodal communicator eager to communicate with partners	Inability to repair communication breakdowns with current AAC strategies resulted in maladaptive behaviors and communication frustration
Increasing receptive language skills	No access to robust vocabulary with current AAC strategies resulted in limited ability to communicate for purposes other than requesting
Emerging recognition of concrete picture symbols	Limited comprehension of abstract picture symbols
Foundational operational competence with high-tech AAC (e.g., activating buttons, navigating between pages)	Raking grasp when interacting with high-tech AAC devices resulting in accidental selections when constructing messages
All members of West's team motivated to implement recommendations	Not yet ambulating independently means device weight and methods of carrying must be considered

However, the iPad-based communication app was ruled out because of the team/family's preference for a dedicated device to support West's understanding of its communicative function, as he perceived the iPad primarily as a leisure tool. Additionally, this app was ruled out due to lack of access to technical support and training (e.g., consultant support, warranty) that is provided with a dedicated device. Ultimately, the features of the dedicated device running the

20-button vocabulary file best matched West's present and future needs and was selected to trial.

Therapeutic Intervention

To ensure that the dedicated device was appropriate for West, a 30-day trial was conducted, led by his private SLP. Data were collected during SLP sessions, ABA sessions, and at home using data collection sheets that captured information on the types of utterances he produced, the purposes for which he communicated (e.g., labeling, requesting, initiating), and the support he required from communication partners to construct utterances (e.g., independently, minimal support with verbal cues, maximal support with physical prompting). To promote West's competence with his device, and increase his communication partners' device skills, a number of goals were targeted across the four areas of communicative competence (Light, 1989), listed below.

1. West will independently navigate at least two levels of his device to request highly preferred items (e.g., foods, shows) in four of five engineered opportunities across three consecutive sessions.
2. West will use his AAC device to label objects and basic concepts (e.g., colors) given fading cues from his communication partners in four of five engineered opportunities across three consecutive sessions.
3. West will protest symbolically using his AAC device given navigation support to the appropriate page from his communication partners and additional cueing in four of five engineered opportunities across three consecutive sessions.
4. West will direct others by creating two-word utterances given a topic display in four of five engineered opportunities across three consecutive sessions.
5. West will fix errors in his messages by restating his message and/or using the clear function given cueing (e.g., verbal cues, modeling) from his communication partner in four of five engineered opportunities across three consecutive sessions.
6. West's communication partners will independently perform at least three functions related to customization and maintenance of West's AAC device (e.g., add button, add page, update software) across three consecutive sessions.

West participated in three 30-minute speech and language therapy sessions per week for the duration of the trial. He also received ABA services four times a week for 30-minute sessions. His AAC device was present and accessible throughout his day and his home communication partners modeled device use continuously. His family members and caregivers quickly adapted to modeling on and programming the device, as well as cueing West while he used it. Due

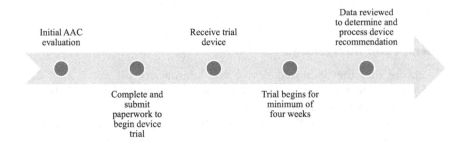

Figure 7.2 Sequence of intervention stages

to consistent therapy access and family support, no adjustments to the intervention were required (Figure 7.2).

Outcomes and Follow-up

When the trial first began, West required modeling from his communication partners to navigate to all areas of his device, as this was his first experience with a category-based AAC device that also utilized predictive linking. He was attentive to modeling and quickly learned to navigate independently to communicate a variety of messages, not only navigating to preferred items (e.g., I want → my stuff→ binky), but also to category folders for concepts he was learning (e.g., describe→ colors; groups→ body).

Another major change noted was the expansion of communicative functions for which West used his device. He previously had only used his AAC device independently to request, requiring physical support from communication partners for other communicative functions (e.g., labeling, protesting). By the end of this trial, West independently requested preferred items using phrases, labeled objects and concepts with single words, and directed the actions of others using two- to three-word utterances in the context of motivating activities. Additionally, West began to use his device for purposes not explicitly targeted, including using his AAC device to engage his brothers in play. Additionally, he learned to state "I need help" to indicate that he couldn't find a word on his device or that the word he needed was not in his device.

In terms of operational competence, West also began to restate incorrect messages made on his AAC device, either independently or with verbal cueing. The clear/delete functions were not present on his previous AAC device, so he required physical support to use this button throughout the trial. A final area of growth was in receptive language. Whereas previously verbal and gestural cues or physical support were required, by the end of the trial he primarily required only verbal cues to alter his message or navigate to a particular area within his device. His family also noted an increased understanding of everyday language used in their household.

West's communication partners demonstrated commitment to teaching him how to use his device (e.g., modeling, fading prompts), and dedication to supporting him by programming his device. His mother was the primary programmer, supported as needed by his private SLP. Over the course of the trial, she learned to add new vocabulary buttons and pages, link these buttons and pages together, hide and color-code buttons, update the software of his vocabulary system and the device itself, and charge the device, among many other skills. She also independently participated in online training through the device company to learn additional features of the device not addressed during therapy sessions.

Due to his success during this trial, West's intervention goals for device use were updated. Revised linguistic competency goals included using two- to three-word combinations to request, direct, and comment; using one word to answer questions; and constructing a variety of syntactic structures (e.g., subject-verb, verb-object). His operational competence goal targeted independent use of the clear function to correct messages with errors. His social competence goals included communicating physical needs, emotional status, and pain/illness to others given prompting, requesting a variety of actions from partners during interactive play, and responding to greetings/partings from others. His revised strategic competence goal emphasized teaching him to protest using symbolic communication (i.e., his AAC device) rather than maladaptive behaviors (e.g., throwing self on ground). This progress is summarized in Table 7.5.

Table 7.5 Summary of Outcomes

Area of Challenge Before Trial	Outcome Post-Trial
• Inability to repair communication breakdowns resulting in maladaptive behaviors and communication frustration	• Learned to ask for help and restate messages with errors using device
	• Significant reduction in maladaptive behaviors and frustration
• Limited ability to communicate for purposes other than requesting due to lack of robust device vocabulary	• Used device to comment, request, engage in play with siblings, and direct the actions of others by the end of the trial
• Limited comprehension of abstract picture symbols	• Learned and independently used several verbs and other abstract symbols (e.g., help) by the end of the trial
• Raking grasp when interacting with high-tech devices resulting in accidental selections	• Acquired full set of keyguards for device to ensure proper support both now and in the future as grid size increases with more advanced vocabulary files
• Not yet ambulating independently	• Increased independence in ambulating over course of trial
	• Communication partners supported West in carrying device from location to location

Complications

One area of complication that arose during the trial related to physical access. Although a customized keyguard was recommended for use throughout the trial, an incorrect keyguard was delivered. This limited West's success with direct selection. Another unit could not be provided, as the trial was only scheduled for a 30-day period. The keyguard was unsuitable for West from motoric and language perspectives. It contained a speech display bar that was only one line wide. The window itself was too narrow for West to access with an isolated digit. Additionally, as a one-line speech display bar only allows for text, he required a multiline speech display bar containing symbol-text combinations so that he could learn new vocabulary by connecting the symbol, text, and speech output, as he did not yet read. Therefore, the keyguard provided was not used during the trial. West was noted to make message errors using an isolated index finger, as his digit slid down the touch screen, accidentally activating incorrect targets. These errors caused noticeable communication frustration. This problem was an immediate area of concern to be addressed when submitting trial data to West's medical insurance company.

Follow-up

West's AAC specialist and OT followed up with his insurance to ensure purchase of the correct keyguard to support access and language interaction. However, given the growth of his language skills during trial, as well as the consideration that this AAC device would need to support his communication needs for some years, the therapists requested a full set of keyguards, one for each vocabulary layout with modifications to the message window opening size, to ensure that physical access would not be a barrier to future progression to larger vocabulary files and grid sizes.

As West's skills with his device continue to progress, his language and motor needs will be assessed on an ongoing basis to ensure his current supports (e.g., vocabulary file, keyguards) continue to meet his needs. These ongoing assessments will allow his team to determine when to advance these supports.

Discussion

This chapter details how the feature-matching process was used to prescribe an AAC device for a young Autistic child. West's growth in competence over the course of the trial is a testament to the importance of a multidisciplinary approach, as many essential features of his device (e.g., keyguard) would have been overlooked if only viewed through the lens of an SLP (Beukelman et al., 2008; Binger et al., 2012; Rose & McMahon, 2018). The communication frustration West experienced from his message errors, caused by physical access difficulties due to lack of a keyguard, further supports this conclusion. Similarly, if the family's desire for a dedicated, rather than integrated, device was not accommodated, the buy-in from his family members could have been affected, increasing the likelihood of device abandonment (Gosnell et al., 2011; Martin & McCormack, 1999; Phillips & Zhao, 1993).

Additionally, targeting device competence using the framework outlined by Light (1989) further contributed to West's progress during the trial. He expanded the communicative functions for which he used the device (linguistic), learned to navigate multiple levels of his device (operational), increased his social interactions with others using the device (social), and learned to restate messages with errors and tell others when he was unable to communicate his message (strategic). His progress was also bolstered by additionally targeting the competence of his communication partners. Teaching West's partners how to program and maintain his device (operational competence) to ensure its functionality for him promoted commitment from his family members and buy-in from West, as their close relationship resulted in his family adding additional, highly-motivating, personalized vocabulary.

This case report illustrates the importance of using the feature-matching process for AAC device selection. By gathering information about West's strengths and challenges in multiple realms, his multidisciplinary team was able to match him with an AAC system whose features matched his current needs and could grow with him. West's success with his new AAC device demonstrates why feature matching continues to be the "gold standard" for AAC device selection.

Client Perspective

West adjusted quickly to his new dedicated AAC device, and returned to using his previous integrated device solely for leisure purposes. He appeared to enjoy having access to a robust vocabulary file in his new device, as evidenced by navigating to various categories within his device and observing the symbols on those pages. He also appeared to enjoy that this device allowed him to communicate with his siblings for social purposes (e.g., calling their names, asking them to play with him). West's family was extremely pleased with the outcome of this process. They noted that observing noticeable changes in West's communication (e.g., reduction in maladaptive behaviors, using his device to socially engage and comment) motivated them to continue consistently implementing the device across environments. His mother independently completed various trainings through the dedicated device company's website to increase her competence with the device (e.g., charging, adding new vocabulary and pages). The family continued to collaborate with his outside providers to ensure that they were able to promote his communication growth as he reached new milestones.

References

Allen, A. A., Schlosser, R. W., Brock, K. L., & Shane, H. C. (2017). The effectiveness of aided augmented input techniques for persons with developmental disabilities: A systematic review. *Augmentative and Alternative Communication, 33*(3), 149–159. doi:10.1080/07434618.2017.1338752

American Occupational Therapy Association. (2014). Occupational therapy practice framework: Domain and process. *American Journal of Occupational Therapy, 68*(1), S1–S48. https://doi.org/10.5014/ajot.2014.682006

Beukelman, D. R., Ball, L. J., & Fager, S. (2008). An AAC personal framework: Adults with acquired complex communication needs. *Augmentative and Alternative Communication, 24*(3), 255–267. https://doi.org/10.1080/07434610802388477

Binger, C., Ball, L., Dietz, A., Kent-Walsh, J., Lasker, J., Lund, S., . . . Quach, W. (2012). Personnel roles in the AAC assessment process. *Augmentative and Alternative Communication, 28*(4), 278–288. https://doi.org/10.3109/07434618.2012.716079

Costello, J., O'Brien, M., & Abramson, J. (2017, September). *Introduction to alternative and augmentative communication.* Presentation during introductory AAC course at the MGH Institute of Health Professions.

Dada, S., Flores, C., Bastable, K., & Schlosser, R. W. (2021). The effects of augmentative and alternative communication interventions on the receptive language skills of children with developmental disabilities: A scoping review. *International Journal of Speech-Language Pathology, 23*(3), 247–257. doi:10.1080/17549507.2020.1797165

Gosnell, J., Costello, J., & Shane, H. (2011). Using a clinical approach to answer, "what communication apps should we use?" *Perspectives on Augmentative and Alternative Communication, 20*(3), 87–96. https://doi.org/10.1044/aac20.3.87

Light, J. (1989). Toward a definition of communicative competence for individuals using alternative and augmentative communication systems. *Augmentative and Alternative Communication, 5*(2), 137–144. https://doi.org/10.1080/07434618912331275126

Light, J., & McNaughton, D. (2014). Communicative competence for individuals who require augmentative and alternative communication: A new definition for a new era of communication? *Augmentative and Alternative Communication, 30*(1), 1–18. https://doi.org/10.3109/07434618.2014.885080

Maljaars, J., Jansen, R., Noens, I., Scholte, E., & van Berckelaer-Onnes, I. (2011). Intentional communication in nonverbal and verbal low-functioning children with autism. *Journal of Communication Disorders, 44*, 601–614. https://doi.org/10.1016/j.jcomdis.2011.07.004

Martin, B., & McCormack, L. (1999). Issues surrounding assistive technology use and abandonment in an emerging technological culture. In C. Bühler & H. Knops (Eds.), *5th European conference for the advancement of assistive technology (AAATE 1999)* (p. 852). IOS Press.

McClintock, K., Hall., S., & Oliver, C. (2003). Risk markers associated with challenging behaviours in people with intellectual disabilities: A meta-analytic study. *Journal of Intellectual Disability Research, 47*, 405–416. https://doi.org/10.1046/j.1365-2788.2003.00517.x

McMahon, L. Buxton, J., & Dellea, P. (2019, January). *OT assessment of AAC: Alternative access technologies & operational competence.* Preconference Presentation at the Assistive Technology Industry Association (ATIA) conference.

Millar, D. C., Schlosser, R., & Light, J. C. (2006). The impact of augmentative and alternative communication intervention on the speech production of individuals with developmental disabilities: A research review. *Journal of Speech, Language, and Hearing Research, 49*(2), 248–264. https://doi.org/10.1044/1092-4388(2006/021)

Phillips, B., & Zhao, H. (1993). Predictors of assistive technology abandonment. *Assistive Technology, 5*(1), 36–45. https://doi.org/10.1080/10400435.1993.10132205

Rose, E., & McMahon, L. (2018, November). *A multidisciplinary approach to AAC: Balancing language, access & function.* Presentation at the American Speech Language Hearing Association (ASHA) convention.

Scherer, M. J., & Galvin, J. C. (1994). Matching people with technology. *Rehab Management, 9,* 128–130.

Schlosser, R. W., & Wendt, O. (2008). Effects of augmentative and alternative communication intervention on speech production in children with autism: A systematic review. *American Journal of Speech-Language Pathology, 17,* 212–230. https://doi.org/10.1044/1058-0360(2008/021)

Sennott, S. C., Light, J. C., & McNaughton, D. (2016). AAC modeling intervention research review. *Research and Practice for Persons with Severe Disabilities, 41,* 101–115. https://doi.org/10.1177/1540796916638822

Shane, H. C., & Costello, J. (1994, November). *Augmentative communication assessment and the feature-matching process.* Mini-seminar presented at the annual convention of the American Speech Language Hearing Association.

Shane, H. C., Laubscher, E., Schlosser, R. W., Flynn, S., Sorce, J. F., & Abramson, J. (2012). Applying technology to visually support language and communication in individuals with ASD. *Journal of Autism and Developmental Disorders, 42,* 1228–1235. https://doi.org/10.1007/s10803-011-1304-z

Sigafoos, J., & Drasgow, E. (2001). Conditional use of aided and unaided AAC: A review and clinical case demonstration. *Focus on Autism and Other Developmental Disabilities, 16*(3), 152–161. https://doi.org/10.1177/108835760101600303

Tager-Flusberg, H., & Kasari, C. (2013). Minimally verbal school-aged children with autism spectrum disorder: The neglected end of the spectrum. *Autism Research, 6*(6), 468–78. https://doi.org/10.1002/aur.1329

Tager-Flusberg, H., Paul, R., & Lord, C. E. (2005). Language and communication in autism. In F. Volkmar, R. Paul, A. Klin, & D. J. Cohen (Eds.), *Handbook of autism and pervasive developmental disorder. 3. Vol. 1.* Wiley. https://doi.org/10.1002/9780470939345.ch12

8 Personal Perspectives on AAC

Gillian Fitzpatrick, Seán Fitzpatrick,
Yvonne Lynch and Martine M. Smith

Introduction

For many individuals, developing competence in using aided communication is an ongoing process that unfolds over extended periods of time. For those with lifelong disabilities such as cerebral palsy, aided communication systems may change and evolve over their entire lifespan. The effects of intervention decisions made in the early preschool years may ripple into adolescence and adulthood, but there are also many decision points along the way, where new directions and new solutions become possible and necessary. Few longitudinal studies have been published (but see Lund & Light, 2006, 2007), but there are a number of personal narratives reflecting on the experience of learning to use aided communication (e.g., Fried-Oken & Bersani, 2000; Pistorius & Davies, 2011), as well as at least one large cross-sectional study *Becoming an Aided Communicator (BAC)*, that explores patterns of language and aided communication use across the age span from 5 to 15 years (von Tetzchner, 2018). These resources highlight the challenge of identifying the optimal communication solution for very young children, often resulting in relatively late provision of aided communication: on average, participants in the BAC study were four years old when aided communication was introduced (von Tetzchner et al., 2018).

The challenges of assessing individuals when many modes of communication are compromised can lead to a failure to recognise the potential for communication and participation, and result in what some individuals experience as wasted years (Pistorius & Davies, 2011). Furthermore, initial systems are often quickly outgrown – on average, participants in the BAC study had used at least three different systems by the time they were seven years old. Changes in an individual's cognitive, linguistic, and motor skills, as well as changes in technology and in environments (e.g., school context) can all trigger reassessment of the match between a communication system and an individual's communication needs (Smith, 2019). Each change can threaten to undermine perceptions of an individual's communicative competence (e.g., Smith et al., 2010). Each new solution demands new learning of all those involved and many new solutions take time to bed down and to become accepted and effective (Alper, 2017; Rackensperger et al., 2005; Singh et al., 2017).

DOI: 10.4324/9781003106739-8

Intervention may extend over many years, even decades, across many settings and life changes. Therapeutic relationships can also extend over long periods, but very often the individuals supporting aided communication interventions change on a regular basis, meaning new relationships must be formed and important information and understandings are vulnerable to being lost and may need to be reconstituted. For most individuals, the one constant across these transitions, disruptions, and changes, remains the family. Family-centred practice is a cornerstone of interventions to support AAC, not only because of the fundamental importance of family relationships but also because of the long-term nature of AAC interventions and the central importance of communication within family systems. Parenting a young person who needs to use aided communication presents many challenges. Parents may encounter expectations that they will be willing and able to take on multiple roles, as parent, carer, therapist, technical support, and as advocate. Parents have commented on the pressures and stresses these multiple demands can pose (e.g., Goldbart & Marshall, 2004; Marshall & Goldbart, 2008). They may find themselves suddenly responsible not only for developing their own technical skills, but also for providing training for other key personnel who interact with their child, often against a backdrop of very limited support (Anderson et al., 2015, 2016). They often provide critical supports for their child through transitions across primary and secondary school settings and into adulthood. They may be the first people to recognise their child's abilities and needs and at times they may face uphill battles in convincing professionals of the validity of their insights. Through all these challenges, they must also juggle the routine demands of parenting, balancing the needs of all members of the family.

This chapter presents the story of Seán, with insights from three key players – Seán himself, his mother, and the speech and language therapist who worked with him over many years. Seán has cerebral palsy and as a result he has limited control of both gross and fine motor skills, requiring adaptations or supports to enable him to carry out most activities. At the time of writing, Seán had completed his mainstream secondary school, and had just completed his final state exams. He had spent the last three months of secondary school working from home due to the restrictions associated with the COVID-19 pandemic. His ambition was to secure a place in a third-level education programme. The structure of this case differs from that of other chapters, as befits the perspectives of the contributors. It is presented as a narrative of recollections by Seán's mother, Seán's comments on the importance of AAC for him, and a description by the therapist of the introduction of AAC and the changes and developments that unfolded over his primary school years.

The therapist first met Seán when he was just over three years old and had no formal communication system. His severe dysarthria and motor difficulties had made it difficult for his parents to find a therapist who could suggest how his communication might be supported. Over the subsequent nine years, Seán learned to use many different aided communication systems and rapidly demonstrated his potential for learning. The therapist's story finishes as Seán transitioned from primary into mainstream secondary school – a major transition for any young person. While Seán continued to avail of SLT supports across the secondary school years with other SLT team members, the early experience of getting access to aided communication was critical in supporting Seán and his family and in laying the foundation for his educational success.

Seán's AAC Journey: A Mother's Perspective

Seán has always been like a sponge, very eager to learn. He loves learning new things. I wanted to give Seán the freedom to choose, to make choices on whatever he wanted in his life. So, first I wanted Seán to learn that he had a choice. This sounds very basic, and it *was* basic to start with. I would hold two things, like books or toys in either hand, and he would look at the one he wanted. I think this was crucial. It gave Seán that sense that he was in the driving seat, not passive. (Seán still makes the majority of decisions in our house today!). At every opportunity, I gave Seán a choice. He got used to choosing for himself, according to his wishes.

The next thing also sounds very basic, but I taught Seán the difference between *yes* and *no*. He began to understand how to express what he wanted or didn't want. I wanted Seán to understand that he could choose whatever path he wanted to in life, that he wasn't passive, letting others make decisions for him. AAC has been an invaluable help in making that happen. Seán could understand what resulted from him choosing this book over that book or by answering yes to a question I asked. Despite not being able to communicate verbally, Seán was still in the driving seat. These two things gave Seán the motivation to express his needs and wants, which is fundamental in any communication.

I think this motivation was very important when it came to using AAC. His first basic communication aid used scan and select with two buttons. Seán understood the basic principle of recognising what he wanted, and after being shown how to achieve this, he went for it! He first tried using switches when he was about three years old. He took to it straight away. He used switches to operate toys or to play a recording of a word or sentence. He quickly learned to use it, pressing a head switch to move through the available symbol or picture options and then pressing a switch on his tray to select the specific symbol he wanted. Eye gaze really made a huge difference to Seán's life. Initially, he was tired but before long he became an expert at it. His 'scan and select' switch system was tiring and slow compared to his eye gaze. When using eye gaze, Seán doesn't have to strain his body to reach switches. On the flip side, it's not instantaneous. There is a time delay between when Seán is asked a question and when he types his response. This is a small price to pay though. I know that Seán wishes it was faster. We have the eye gaze set at a two-second dwell time on a particular letter or character (meaning that a letter is selected only after Seán has maintained a gaze on it for two seconds).

Key People as Supports

There were a number of people over the years who were important in helping us to ensure Seán's needs were met. Yvonne (SLT), who was based in a clinic in Dublin, gave us a lot of support. She was involved with Seán when he was young. We were so relieved and excited to meet her. I found her input invaluable because, unfortunately, there was a lack of expertise in AAC locally. Yvonne could see what we already knew about Seán – that he had lots of potential and she was very encouraging. We looked forward to every session with Yvonne. We were excited about giving Seán the very best chance to unlock his potential and we did this together, as a team.

Alan of Enable Ireland gave us a lot of technical support, and he was involved with Seán from a young age also. Nick from a company based in the UK demonstrated how eye gaze could work for Seán. After his initial demonstration we were blown away, I could see how eye gaze could have a huge impact on Seán's life. Nick set up the eye gaze for Seán and the company in the UK provided support over the phone or by email.

There have also been a few special needs assistants and teachers who have embraced the use of eye gaze in the classroom. This gives us as parents great peace of mind. We know that Seán will use his eye gaze and not become frustrated that it is not set up for him properly. (Some assistants and teachers we have encountered along our journey have been frightened or sceptical of this technology, which doesn't help). We also had a training day for Seán's teachers and special needs assistants, which I think is vital.

Key Elements in Seán's Success

Literacy

I definitely think that having a literacy-based system over a symbol-based one was a huge motivational factor for Seán. Seán never showed much interest in symbols, but the written word really captured his attention. We used symbols when he was young. We had symbols stuck on doorways and on the sink, beside toy boxes and all around the house, and we used symbols in a folder in playschool. Importantly, Seán has always had a hard copy, a folder or laminated chart of symbols, including the alphabet, as a back-up to his technology. As far as I can remember, Seán was three years old when we introduced the alphabet to him. He quickly moved on to spelling words and forming sentences and he could spell lots of three-letter words by the time he started school. The laminator and rolls of Velcro were our allies back in the day!

I know there are symbol-based systems that work well but Seán was drawn to the written word. It has given him the freedom to express himself without being limited to a symbol.

There just aren't symbols for certain things you would like to express. Seán will attempt to spell words that are difficult for him to spell rather than sticking to words he knows and uses regularly. It allows him to be very clear and precise in the message he wants to convey.

Eye Gaze Access

Seán's eye gaze has been invaluable to him in the context of his social life. He has a lot of questions to ask, and he can ask them all thanks to his device. He has been able to congratulate a friend on graduating from university, or to congratulate a Gaelic footballer[1] on receiving his All Stars award.[2] This is where a literacy-based system is key. (How could he even attempt to convey that using a symbol-based system of communication?). The delight on his face when someone responds to his communication is something I will always treasure. Funnily enough, lately, if I give Seán the option of using his device or not he will say *no* to using it. He says that he misses a lot in the conversation. He misses the eye contact and facial and body language that can convey so much. I think the device itself blocks his view too.

AAC and Education

AAC really comes into its own in the educational setting. Using AAC and, in particular, his eye gaze has enabled Seán to participate not only in the classroom with his peers but also in state exams. Systems have changed over the years. Seán was using a scan-and-select system with a motion pad in primary school. He scanned using a small button/switch on his head rest and he selected the letter or number with a switch that was attached onto his tray with Velcro. The scan-and-select method worked well but it was tiring for Seán. We tried attaching an eye gaze camera onto his motion pad first, but it wasn't until he got the GridPad™ with an inbuilt camera that things really took off.

Now, Seán can do his schoolwork and either email it to his teacher or print it out either at school or at home. He can browse the internet. He can participate in the classroom by answering a question or he can volunteer some information. Seán completed his Junior Certificate (a state examination that students typically take after four years in secondary school) and did very well using his eye gaze. He typed the answers using his eye gaze access system and he had a scribe who wrote his answers down on the paper for him. He did his Leaving Certificate Applied (the final state exam at the end of secondary school) and completed lots of tasks and projects using his eye gaze. It has been and is an invaluable tool in his educational journey.

AAC and the Future

Seán is doing a Post-Leaving Certificate (PLC) course in a local college to earn points to apply for a third-level course at Galway-Mayo Institute of Technology (in Ireland, entrance to third-level programmes is competitive and based on points achieved in the Leaving Certificate examination and/or a PLC course).

He did his interview online using Zoom™ and answered questions using his eye gaze system.

Seán will always use technology to aid in his communication. His eye gaze system is probably due an upgrade soon so I will contact the suppliers in this regard. I've no doubt (this company) are at the forefront in delivering the latest technology to those who need AAC.

Seán's View on His Experience with AAC

I have a device which I control with my eyes. This is called an eye gaze. Anyone can use it, but I am very fast at using this device. I use my eye gaze in school when I'm doing my school work and projects, etc. If I didn't have my eye gaze I would be devastated. Before I got my eye gaze I used a device called a motion pad and I used two switches. One switch was used by my head and another was used by my hand. I scanned the keyboard with my head switch and selected the character with my hand switch. We tried using an eye gaze camera that plugged into my motion pad. It wasn't anything like my GridPad with inbuilt cameras. I found the switches very slow and I always got tired using it. I find my eye gaze is very quick and fast to use and it makes my life easier and I'm less tired. I started using my current eye gaze system when I was in second year and I did my Junior Cert using my eye gaze. I think that eye gaze would be better for those who need a device like me; for example, if you want to understand someone who is having difficulties saying a word. My advice is to start using eye gaze early, it would be easier for them to talk. And I think it's worth considering that special needs assistants all need training on how to mount the device.

The Speech and Language Therapist Perspective

Background Information

Seán was three years old when he was referred to the clinic for an AAC assessment. He attended with both his parents for a joint speech and language therapy and occupational therapy assessment. His parents reported that he appeared to understand what they said. He had been assessed by a psychologist who had limited experience with children with physical disabilities. On the basis of that assessment, the psychologist reported his cognitive function was at a nine-month level. Seán's parents reported that he was seeing a speech and language therapist locally who had recommended an iTalk2™ communication aid (see www.ablenetinc.com/italk2/). Seán was also seeing a speech and language therapist privately who was working on nonspeech oral motor exercises to try and support Seán to develop speech. Seán's mother felt a focus on communication would be better for Seán than persisting with speech exercises.

In the assessment, Seán presented as alert and he engaged with a range of activities. He had some control of his hands, but access was effortful and he was very frustrated by not being able to communicate what he wanted. Seán demonstrated understanding of using a switch for cause-effect activities. He was able to make nondirected choices in activities from a choice of four photographs (for example, when singing "Old MacDonald had a Farm", Seán was asked to select which animal to sing about next, and he made a choice from photos of a cow, horse, goat, and pig). He was also able to make directed choices where there was a correct answer in activities (e.g., "Now let's sing about the cow, can you find me the cow?"). He had the ability to sustain attention for extended periods of time and was highly engaged in all presented activities. While able to demonstrate the ability to make choices from a choice of four, Seán was not able to consistently use the iTalk2 (www.inclusive.co.uk/italk2-communication-aid-p2082) due to physical challenges bringing his hands to the buttons and moving between the two buttons. Seán was given an opportunity to use two switches to access a computer with switch-controlled games. The occupational therapist held one switch near Seán's head and the second switch was placed on his tray. He demonstrated immediate understanding and the ability to control two switches. At the end of the appointment, Seán's parents asked the team if they felt he had potential. As parents, they felt he did, but they had not been given hope by previous professionals. We agreed that Seán indeed had enormous potential.

Our first priorities for Seán were to provide him with ways of controlling his environment and making choices on a daily basis. Our sense was that he would progress rapidly, and he needed a system as soon as possible. We also felt he had the potential to outgrow systems quickly. We began with a low-tech system of photos and symbols focused on giving Seán control and choices across the day. Simultaneously, we worked on two-switch stepped scanning to provide Seán with a consistent and reliable way to control a communication aid. In stepped scanning, pressing one switch moves through the available options, the person stops pressing the moving switch when they reach the item they want and then they press a second switch to choose that item. The aim was to develop communication and operational skills in parallel, while giving Seán immediate control of his environment.

Intervention

Seán progressed very quickly with AAC, but the priorities identified in that first appointment (autonomy and control) continued across the primary school years. There was also an ongoing tension between balancing the need to support Seán's rapid language learning and expressive needs with the challenges he experienced in accessing his communication systems. This balance was achieved through close collaboration with Seán and his family.

Journey with Language

Seán progressed quickly from symbol choices to an engineered environment (i.e., presentation of symbols throughout the environment) with topic boards using core vocabulary, to a robust language system on a dedicated device, through to a literacy-based system. In addition, there was an increasing focus on using his own natural speech. At all stages, the goal was to try and keep up with Seán and his voracious need for more language to express himself and engage in his school, family, and community life.

Physical Access

Seán took to two-switch scanning very quickly and was fast and accurate using this method. However, switch use was effortful for Seán; at the end of a therapy session, he was often damp with sweat from the physical effort of communicating. His physiotherapist also had concerns about the longer-term musculoskeletal effects of switch use on his neck. Throughout Seán's childhood the focus was on trying to reduce the effort and maximise the efficiency of access to communication, while maintaining his physical abilities and consistent and accurate access. For example, when Seán was using two-switch stepped scanning in school, work continued on using low-tech systems with eye- or fist-pointing at other times in the day. These access methods were less independent (i.e., Seán needed the support of a communication partner) but they were also less effortful so he could maintain his energy levels across the day.

Seán's progress was constant, and often rapid. As outlined in the timeline (see Table 8.1), he transitioned across multiple systems and tried many different access methods over the years. Each new system or access method required new learning, not just of Seán but also of his family and all those supporting him. A key concern was ensuring that Seán's development was not constrained by systems provided for him, meaning there was a need for constant review and monitoring to ensure changes were identified and implemented as quickly as possible.

Collaborative Relationship

Working with Seán and his family was always about listening to what they had to say and providing options for them to consider and identify what was best for them as a family. When he was very young, Seán's parents recognised he had potential and that a focus on communication development was needed – something that they felt was missed by a number of professionals, resulting in their feeling that they were not being listened to.

Families as Experts

As in many aspects of intervention involving AAC, there were often several possibilities that could work for Seán; at each point, it was important to be clear on what was the best fit in that particular context. Decisions were made through discussion. Often Gillian and Seán were provided with a number of

Table 8.1 Timeline

Initial assessment 3 years, 6 months	**Provide control and choice while building AAC skills** • E-Tran frame™ and photos • 2-switch scanning games
4 years	**Sean demonstrated rapid progression with language while access remained very effortful** • Photo choices –> topic organised folder of 2" PCS symbols • E-Tran frame™ frame with up to 4 symbols • Moving to fist pointing to 6 symbols • Predominance of nouns • Sibling board for play activities • Continued ++ effort for access • Use of BIGmack
5–6 years	**Language developing** • Symbol-based category board • Greater emphasis on core vocabulary • Switch to syntactic board • Focus on developing literacy and modeling multisymbol utterances and strategic use of symbols • Assessed by psychologist with experience of physical disability (in average range)
6 years	**More independent AAC use** • Dynavox V with Gateway 40™ • 2-switch step scanning • Sean spent a lot of time searching for vocabulary to say what he wanted. An intervention programme was put in place to support strategic use of vocabulary and to also reduce search efforts.
10 years	• Technical difficulties with the device • Moving away from using symbols – preference for literacy • Emergence of spoken language – large single-word vocabulary • Use of texting on iPhone and iPad • Returned to using a Dynavox 3100™ with an alphabet grid only • Matching board put in place
11 years	• Family purchased iPad – direct access with typing • Multidisciplinary assessment with occupational therapy, physiotherapy, speech and language therapy, Sean, and his family to consider, discuss, and plan long-term access for communication that would maintain Sean's physical function. • Exploring new device options • C10™ trial –> Sean learned quickly how to control an eye gaze system. Sean and his family felt it was a very useful tool but not for communication at this time. They felt the loss of eye contact impacted too much on communication interaction. Agreed to implement an eye gaze system for academic work but not for communication. • Motionpad™ loan
12 years	• ISAAC summer camp and conference • Realisation of the need for quickfire vocabulary • Access constraints – There was a need for a layout that can facilitate hand access, 2-switch step scan, and potentially eye gaze for academic work.

options and together the advantages and disadvantages were discussed. Gillian and Seán always made the final decision. Sometimes, they found their own solutions to different challenges, and it was important to recognise what worked for them and to build on their problem solving. For example, at one appointment, Gillian reported that Seán had started texting on her iPhone so we looked at this in the session. We discussed how he could use texting and also identified other opportunities to use and develop his literacy skills. This shared decision making meant appointments did not always go as planned; however, it was important to actively listen to Gillian and Seán, and to be flexible in the direction taken in assessment and intervention. Sometimes that meant saying in appointments, *I'll need to think about how we can make that work* or *I'll need to find out more information about that.* Decision making was shared and therefore give-and-take was needed on all sides.

AAC in the Context of the Family

While physical access to a device was an ongoing concern and discussion point when working with Seán and his family, the first priority was to support Seán to communicate and develop language. Because of this focus and prioritisation, Seán went on to develop language, literacy, and communication competencies. As a result, it was possible to find technological solutions to different challenges along the way, solutions that complemented his linguistic and communication skills. Sometimes in planning interventions to support AAC, there is a focus on sorting access first, but this can mean that vital language learning opportunities are lost. It is important that language learning and building communication competencies are addressed first.

Summary and Conclusions

The three perspectives shared in this chapter highlight some of the challenges that young people and their families encounter as they bring AAC into their homes and lives. Across the three accounts, there are some common themes. One is the importance of early intervention, so that motivation to communicate can be supported and can drive the effort needed to develop skills. A second is the value of listening to and working with families to find solutions that fit the needs of everyone involved. A third theme is the importance of constantly reviewing systems and access methods, to ensure that language learning needs are met in a way that is physically acceptable. This vigilance requires constant engagement on the part of professionals working in this area, to ensure they are aware of new developments. Seán's mother points out that, despite extraordinary innovations, technological solutions can sometimes present new barriers – the loss of eye contact and access to facial expression that has recently led Seán to opt not to use his high-tech system in conversations with peers. This point highlights the importance of ensuring that there is always another option available – whether through low-tech systems or using unaided communication modes. A fourth theme that emerges is the importance of key coworkers. In this instance, a small number of people were pivotal in supporting the family across many years and many changes. The opportunity to maintain contact with key supports across transitions can be invaluable in maintaining important knowledge about a service user but also in supporting families. Finally, both Seán's mother and the SLT highlight the importance of supporting language, literacy, and communication as the starting point. Even complex, innovative systems such as eye gaze access are simply tools. Without the raw materials of language and communication, their value will always be limited.

Notes

1 Gaelic football is a uniquely Irish form of football that is played between two teams of 15 players on a grass pitch.
2 All Stars awards are awarded annually by the Gaelic Athletic Association-Gaelic Players' Association to the best player in each of the 15 playing positions to create a special team of the year. These awards are highly prized.

References

Alper, M. (2017). *Giving voice: Mobile communication, disability and inequality.* The MIT Press.

Anderson, K., Balandin, S., & Stancliff, R. (2015). Alternative service delivery models for families with a new speech generating device: Perspectives of parents and therapists. *International Journal of Speech-Language Pathology, 17,* 185–195. http://dx.doi.org.elib.tcd.ie/10.3109/17549507.2014.979876

Anderson, K., Balandin, S., & Stancliff, R. (2016). "It's got to be more than that". Parents and speech-language pathologists discuss training content for families with a new speech generating device. *Assistive Technology, 11,* 375–384. www.dx.doi.org.elib.tcd.ie/10.3109/17483107.2014.967314

Fried-Oken, M., & Bersani, H. (2000). *Speaking up and spelling it out: Personal essays on augmentative and alternative communication.* Paul Brookes Publishing Co.

Goldbart, J., & Marshall, J. (2004). "Pushes and pulls" on the parents of children who use AAC. *Augmentative and Alternative Communication, 20*(4), 194–200.

Lund, S. K., & Light, J. (2006). Long-term outcomes for individuals who use augmentative and alternative communication: Part I – what is a "good" outcome? *Augmentative and Alternative Communication, 22*(4), 284–299.

Lund, S. K., & Light, J. (2007). Long term outcomes for individuals who use AAC: Part II – expressive communication. *Augmentative and Alternative Communication, 23,* 1–15.

Marshall, J., & Goldbart, J. (2008). 'Communication is everything I think.' Parenting a child who needs augmentative and alternative communication (AAC). *International Journal of Language and Communication Disorders, 43*(1), 77–98. doi:10.1080/13682820701267444

Pistorius, M., & Davies, M. L. (2011). *Ghost boy.* Simon & Schuster.

Rackensperger, T., Krezman, C., McNaughton, D., Williams, M. B., & D'Silva, K. (2005). "When I first got it, I wanted to throw it off a cliff": The challenges and benefits of learning AAC technologies as described by adults who use AAC. *Augmentative and Alternative Communication, 21*(3), 165–186.

Singh, S., Hussein, N., Kamal, R., & Hassan, H. (2017). Reflections of Malaysian parents of children with developmental disabilities on their experiences with AAC. *Augmentative and Alternative Communication, 33*(2), 110–120. doi:10.1080/07434618.2017.1309457

Smith, M. (2019). Innovations for supporting communication: Opportunities and challenges for people with complex communication needs. *Folia Phoniatrica et Logopedia, 71,* 156–167. doi:10.1159/000496729

Smith, M., Murray, J., von Tetzchner, S., & Langan, P. (2010). A tale of transitions: The challenges of integrating speech synthesis in aided communication. In J. Mullenix & S. Stern (Eds.), *Computer synthesized speech technologies: Tools for aiding impairment* (pp. 234–256). IGI Global.

von Tetzchner, S. (2018). Introduction to the special issue on aided language processes, development, and use: An international perspective. *Augmentative and Alternative Communication, 34*(1), 1–15. doi:10.1080/07434618.2017.1422020

von Tetzchner, S., Launonen, K., Batarowicz, B., d'Oliveira de Paula Nunes, L. R., Walter, C., Oxley, J., . . . Deliberato, D. (2018). Communication aid provision and use among children and adolescents developing aided communication: An international survey. *Augmentative and Alternative Communication, 34*(1), 79–91. doi:10.1080/07434618.2017.1422019

9 Augmentative and Alternative Communication for People with Aphasia

Michelle Kryc and Aimee Dietz

Introduction

AAC includes various modalities of communication that facilitate and enhance a person's ability to make requests and comments, ask questions, and complete other daily functions of communication. AAC strategies and tools are categorized as either aided or unaided. The benefits of low-tech AAC (Garrett, 1989; Rose, 2013) and high-tech AAC for people with aphasia (Dietz et al., 2020; Taylor et al., 2019) have been confirmed. This case report focuses on the use of high-technology AAC, specifically mobile technology and communication applications (apps), for a person with aphasia.

Aphasia is an acquired language disorder that is often a result of a brain injury in the left hemisphere (American Speech–Language–Hearing Association, 2020a) and can affect all forms of language, including verbal expression, written expression, reading comprehension, and auditory comprehension, to varying degrees of severity. Although linguistic skills are heavily impacted in aphasia, other cognitive functions typically remain relatively intact, such as autobiographical memory, visual-spatial processing, and facial recognition (Beukelman et al., 2015). These strengths can be harnessed to promote the successful use of AAC technologies with people with aphasia. Nonetheless, AAC is often not considered in the acute or subacute phase of post-stroke aphasia rehabilitation until traditional restorative interventions have been exhausted; however, some researchers suggest that early AAC intervention, "may yield widespread positive effects" (Dietz et al., 2020, p. 4). As such, this case report aims to highlight how recent advances in technology, such as the iPad and iPhone, have created a more socially acceptable option that is financially and operationally accessible for people with aphasia (McNaughton & Light, 2013).

These technological innovations have provided people with aphasia with several AAC app options; however, it is imperative to consider the unique profile of each person with aphasia. That is, one app *does not* fit all. To best evaluate each person with aphasia, a feature matching assessment is required. Feature matching is the systematic process of pairing an individual with an AAC system tailored to their strengths and weaknesses,

DOI: 10.4324/9781003106739-9

to best fit their current and future communicative needs (Gosnell et al., 2011). The effective use of feature matching and available AAC assessment tools can create a more positive relationship between person and device, ultimately increasing AAC acceptance and decreasing device abandonment (Binger et al., 2012). Throughout this case report, the speech–language pathologist (SLP) illustrates the successful combination of traditional and AAC-focused treatment approaches to facilitate and restore communication. This is in harmony with the benefits of a multimodal communication training program as described in the literature (Purdy & Van Dyke, 2011; Wallace et al., 2014). For this case report, a multimodal approach included incorporating high-tech AAC alongside various traditional restorative language therapies.

Patient Information

Lucy, a 57-year-old female, survived a left middle cerebrovascular accident approximately 10 months prior to this case report. She lives at home with Jim, her husband of 25 years. They have two daughters, aged 23 and 21, both of whom live away from home on their respective college campuses. Lucy is a secretary at a local law firm, where she organizes schedules, maintains the firm's website, answers phone calls, and manages other administrative duties. This position requires Lucy to use the computer daily and communicate frequently with clients. Lucy uses Facebook to maintain relationships with friends and family. She has the word prediction function enabled on her iPhone, which assists with texting and messaging on Facebook. Jim reports that when Lucy attempts to make a request, comment, or question verbally, she is often unable to "get a word out" and occasionally "shuts down." Jim notes that she often points when she is having difficulty speaking and becomes frustrated when others do not understand. He says that she is most successful with verbal communication when she is with familiar people such as friends and family or when using pictures on her phone or on Facebook. Lucy enjoys gardening and spending time with her family and friends, although her husband mentioned that she hasn't seen her friends in months. Quality time with family and friends remains a priority for Lucy and her family.

Clinical Findings

Case History

Upon arrival at the hospital, Lucy was experiencing numbness and weakness in her right upper extremities and right facial droop. Her attending doctors ordered a speech-language pathology evaluation to examine her speech, language, and swallow function. The SLP began with an oral mechanism examination (OME), where she observed slight right-sided asymmetry, along with

Table 9.1 Timeline of Assessment

April 17, 2019: Lucy was admitted to the hospital following symptoms of right-sided tingling and weakness, slurred speech, and right-sided facial droop. The neurologist viewed the CT scan and reported an infarct in the anterior portion of the frontal lobe near Brodmann's area 44. A modified barium swallow study (MBSS) indicated moderate residue in the valleculae.

April 22, 2019: Lucy was discharged from the hospital and referred to an inpatient rehabilitation facility where the SLP administered several assessments, including the *Western Aphasia Battery-Revised* (Kertesz, 2006) to better understand Lucy's communicative status. A repeat MBSS was completed, with no concerns regarding residue.

April 22–May 1, 2019: Traditional restorative language treatment began. The SLP completed an AAC assessment.

May 1, 2019: Lucy's family decided to purchase an iPad to begin AAC implementation.

May 2, 2019: Lucy was provided with the Tobii Dynavox® Snap + Core First™ application.

May 3, 2019: A dual therapy approach was utilized to facilitate communication. The clinician used personally relevant information in both the traditional language therapy and the structured AAC treatment.

June 27, 2019: Lucy was discharged from the inpatient rehabilitation facility and followed up with an outpatient SLP to continue practice with AAC.

---

right-sided labial weakness. Notably, no tongue weakness was reported. Next, the SLP conducted an informal language evaluation, which revealed deficits in spoken language expression, along with mild dysarthria and probable mild verbal apraxia. The SLP also reported that Lucy's receptive skills were functional for basic interactions, stating that she was successfully able to follow two-step directions. High-level comprehension skills were not assessed at this time. The SLP ordered and completed a modified barium swallow study (MBSS) to examine the integrity of Lucy's swallow. The study revealed moderate residue in the valleculae that was eliminated with multiple swallows and liquid wash. Because the clinician was confident of Lucy's cognitive capabilities, she placed Lucy on a regular diet, with instruction to take small bites and alternate solids and liquids. The clinician saw Lucy throughout her stay to work on spoken expression and strengthening her swallow mechanism. After five days in the hospital, Lucy was transferred to an inpatient rehabilitation center for more intensive treatment.

Speech-Language and Swallowing Assessment

At the inpatient rehabilitation facility, the SLP began with a traditional aphasia assessment, a key step prior to the AAC assessment due to the unique profile of needs associated with different aphasias. The AAC assessment is a multifactorial process that involves more than AAC selection. Several cognitive, linguistic, and ecological considerations must be reviewed. The clinician modeled Lucy's AAC assessment after the AAC assessment procedures recommended by the American Speech-Language-Hearing

Association (see www.asha.org/practice-portal/professional-issues/augmentative-and-alternative-communication/#collapse_1).

Self-Report and Ecological Inventory

The SLP conducted an informal interview with Lucy and Jim to get a better understanding of life prior to Lucy's stroke. Lucy then completed the *Stroke and Aphasia Quality of Life Scale-39 (SAQOL-39)* (Hilari et al., 2003) with occasional comprehension support from the SLP. The SAQOL-39 examines four domains: physical, psychosocial, communication, and energy. This patient reported outcome measure uses two nominal scales starting from "1 = *couldn't do at all*" to "5 = *no trouble at all*" and "1 = *definitely yes*" to "5 = *definitely no.*" The higher the score the better the quality of life. Lucy received a mean score of 2.6/5, a communication score of 2/5, a physical score of 2.8/5, and a psychosocial score of 2/5.

This scale opens the opportunity for the SLP to ask follow-up questions on stimuli that yielded low scores. Using the SAQOL-39 as a guide and motivational interviewing, the patient and SLP can identify intervention goals. It is important to include the co-survivor during this process. The goals generated should be personally relevant and functional to increase motivation. Lucy's communication goals were to talk with her daughters about gardening, their college experiences, and other family-related topics.

Next, Lucy and Jim completed the *Communicative Effectiveness Index (CETI)* (Lomas et al., 1989). The purpose of this index is to better understand the caregiver's perception of their loved one's current communicative abilities. The clinician adapted this tool so that Lucy could also report her opinion of her communication skills, which was central to her taking an active role in the rehabilitation process. This is a Visual Analogue scale questionnaire that includes questions about the patient's ability to respond in different communication situations. Answers range from "*not at all able*" to "*as able as before.*" The patient draws a line to represent where they feel they "fit" on the scale. The clinician then measures the distance from "not at all able" to obtain a numerical value. Discrepancies in answers may arise between caregivers and the individual with aphasia; thus, it is important that they complete the index separately. Both Jim and Lucy had similar results.

Language Assessment

The SLP used the *Western Aphasia Battery-Revised (WAB-R)* (Kertesz, 2006) to gain an overall appreciation of Lucy's aphasia type and severity. Her profile was consistent with Broca's aphasia and her score of 61.9 indicated a moderate severity. Her spoken language was telegraphic and consisted mostly of content words (e.g., concrete nouns such as 'table' and 'shirt') in response to the picture description task; however, she used some meaningful phrases. Table 9.2 summarizes her performance on the WAB-R. The writing portions

Table 9.2 Summary of Lucy's Performance on the Western Aphasia Battery-Revised (Kertesz, 2006)

WAB-R SUBTESTS	TOTAL POINTS	LUCY'S POINTS
SPONTANEOUS SPEECH		
Fluency, grammatical competence, and paraphasias	10	5
Information content	10	4
Spontaneous Speech Total	*20*	*9*
AUDITORY VERBAL COMPREHENSION		
Yes/no questions	60	42
Auditory word recognition	60	50
Sequential commands	80	67
Auditory Verbal Comprehension Total	*200*	*159*
REPETITION		
Repetition Total	100	77
NAMING & WORD FINDING		
Object naming	60	45
Word fluency	20	6
Sentence completion	10	7
Responsive speech	10	5
Total	*100*	*63*
APHASIA QUOTIENT	*100*	*61.9*

of the WAB-R and other supplemental sections revealed that her written language mimicked her spoken expression. However, the reading section indicated that reading comprehension was a strength, compared to auditory comprehension.

Sensory and Motor Status

A follow-up MBSS was completed and revealed an improvement in Lucy's laryngeal strength and valving with no residue in the valleculae. The SLP administered the *Scanning/Visual Field/Print Size/Attention Screening Task* (Garret & Lasker, 2007d; https://cehs.unl.edu/aac/aphasia-assessment-materials/) to identify appropriate visual accommodations for Lucy. This screening tool suggested that Lucy did not have visual field deficits (confirmed by occupational therapy) and was able to identify written text using 12-point font. A pure tone audiological hearing screening identified normal hearing. The physical and occupational therapists (PT/OT) at the inpatient rehabilitation centre treated Lucy's right-sided upper extremity numbness and weakness.

AAC Assessment

Based on the results of the WAB-R (Kertesz, 2006), sensory and motor status, and patient needs findings, the SLP decided that restorative treatment should focus on enhancing semantic networks and increasing syntactic complexity. A hybrid approach to treatment was implemented to optimize overall communicative effectiveness (Wallace & Kayode, 2017), on the basis that Lucy would receive maximal effect if these traditional treatments were offered in conjunction with an AAC intervention designed to meet the restorative goals. The results of the CETI (Lomas et al., 1989) and the SAQOL-39 (Hilari et al., 2003) indicated that Lucy's current communicative abilities were not being met by verbal output alone. The SLP suggested AAC as a restorative treatment approach and communicative support for Lucy. After reflecting on this information, and with input from their daughters, Lucy and Jim agreed that this would be a good avenue to explore while on the inpatient rehab unit.

The SLP first completed the *AAC-Aphasia Categories of Communicators Checklist* (Garret & Lasker, 2007a; https://cehs.unl.edu/aac/aphasia-assessment-materials/). This checklist identifies communicator types based on their abilities and needs. Individuals are broadly categorized as either partner-dependent communicators or independent communicators. Partner-dependent communicators rely more heavily on someone to assist them with communication; in contrast, independent communicators do not.

The SLP observed Lucy interacting with Jim and with other inpatients during recreational therapy; she also interviewed Lucy alone and together with Jim. When Lucy and Jim were together, Jim often did most of the communication. During one mealtime observation, Lucy became frustrated when Jim was unable to decipher her intended message. In another instance, when Lucy misplaced her cell phone, she was able to gain Jim's attention and communicate this using gestures and telegraphic phrases. In conversation with unfamiliar communication partners, such as the other patients and nurses, Lucy often turned to Jim to clarify or expand her messages. In these situations, Jim answered questions for Lucy and Lucy responded by nodding in agreement. One morning, Lucy was conversing with another patient about their family life. In this interaction, the SLP noted that Lucy appeared more comfortable and was able to produce some meaningful utterances when talking about her daughters. Additionally, during a therapy session, Lucy confidently greeted her PT and OT and answered basic messages such as, "how are you?" In the individual interview, the SLP provided Lucy with images and a QWERTY communication board to augment her spoken expression. Lucy was able to answer a few personal questions and wrote down her street name when asked to provide her address. Lucy did not initiate any questions of her own. In the interview with Jim, Jim reported that he often communicated for Lucy because she "just gets so frustrated." He said that he understood Lucy's spoken expression or her intended message about 70% of the time, but that his daughters only understood 50% of the time. After this observation, Lucy was classified as a dependent communicator, specifically a transitional communicator (see Table 9.3).

Table 9.3 Summary of Lucy's Strengths and Challenges as a Transitional Communicator (Garrett & Lasker, 2007a)

STRENGTHS *of a Transitional Communicator*	CHALLENGES *of a Transitional Communicator*
"can initiate a partial message on occasion and in specific contexts, but requires support to communicate a complete message"	*"unable to repair conversation breakdowns independently"*
"can request by pointing or vocalizing"	*"does not initiate questions, but may initiate requests for physical needs or comment without cues"*
"can greet or produce gestural or spoken word responses in automatic social conversation"	*"uses mostly automatic speech, if any"*

The *AAC-Aphasia Categories of Communicators Checklist* (Garret & Lasker, 2007a; https://cehs.unl.edu/aac/aphasia-assessment-materials/) provided the clinician with an outline of Lucy's current strengths and needs regarding her ability to utilize AAC. Specifically, she learned that the treatment plan should include strategies to switch communication modalities to address communication breakdowns. In addition, this checklist provided preliminary information regarding Lucy's ability to navigate through an AAC board, suggesting further testing was warranted to assess this skill (see the section on "Cognitive Communication Assessment").

Social Communication Assessment

The *Aphasia Needs Assessment* (Garrett & Lasker, 2007b; https://cehs.unl.edu/aac/aphasia-assessment-materials/) is a questionnaire that helps clinicians appreciate current communication demands and desires. It includes probes regarding the person's perceived communication needs and abilities across a variety of communication environments and partners. The assessment requires individuals to place a checkmark in boxes they feel are relevant to their personal situation. For example, in response to a question, "*What communication skills are most difficult for you?*" an individual can choose from options such as, "*getting someone's attention, introducing myself and others, engaging in "small talk"* . . . *etc.*" (Garret & Lasker, 2007b). To promote independent completion of the tool, without help from her husband, the clinician modified the *Aphasia Needs Assessment* to be consistent with aphasia-friendly principles such as enlarged and boldened font, increased white space (Rose et al., 2012), and photos (Dietz et al., 2009). Table 9.4 displays key findings from the assessment.

Cognitive Communication Assessment

A subtest of the *Cognitive Linguistic Quick Test (CLQT)* (Helm-Estabrooks, 2001) was used to assess cognitive flexibility. There is evidence that the Symbol

Table 9.4 Key Findings from the Aphasia Needs Assessment (Garrett & Lasker, 2007b; https://cehs.unl.edu/aac/aphasia-assessment-materials/)

Probe	Lucy's Responses
"Which situations give you the most difficulty with communication?"	1. *Talking on the phone* 2. *Conversations with family or friends* 3. *Conversations with strangers* 4. *Doctor/medical settings*
"What would you like to talk about during conversations"	1. *Funny stories about our children* 2. *Current events* 3. *Hobbies or unique interests* 4. *Favorite meals/restaurants* 5. *My stroke and/or other medical issues*
"Which communication skills are the most difficult for you?"	1. *Engaging in "small talk"* 2. *Introducing myself and others* 3. *Explaining about aphasia and how I communicate* 4. *Spelling*
"Do you do most of the communicating yourself"	*No*
"If you answered "no," who does?"	*Jim*
"What kind of materials would you like to read?"	1. *Daily newspapers*

Trails subtest of the CLQT (Helm-Estabrooks, 2001) is a reliable tool to assess the ability to navigate through different AAC interface designs, for example, to navigate from a superordinate folder on a grid display (food) to a button within this folder (apple) (Wallace et al., 2010). Initially, Lucy struggled with this task; however, she responded well to instruction and modeling, suggesting that she likely had the cognitive flexibility to navigate through AAC interface pages with focused instruction.

Symbol Assessment

High-tech AAC devices offer different representations of communication. Some use iconic symbols to represent a word while others use personally relevant photographs. To provide Lucy with the most appropriate AAC system, the *Multimodal Communication Screening Test for People with Aphasia (MCST-A)* (Garret & Lasker, 2007c; https://cehs.unl.edu/aac/ aphasia-assessment-materials/) was administered to determine (1) how efficiently and effectively Lucy used AAC strategies to respond to specific communicative situations, and (2) to identify what type of symbol system might serve Lucy best.

The SLP gave Lucy the MCST-A stimulus book, which contains various message representation options, such as line drawings, symbols, photographs, and an alphabet board to use as communicative supports. Next, the SLP asked the stimulus questions provided in the MCST-A scoring form. For example,

"How can you tell me where you live?" "Which state do you live in?" (Garret & Lasker, 2007c). Lucy's response was as follows:

A. *Pointed to the location on the map on p. 5.*
B. *Pointed to the first letter of city name on alphabet page.*
C. *Partially spelled city/town name*

During the assessment, Lucy utilized symbols to relay information (e.g., pointing to a shoe to suggest she needed shoes) and demonstrated the ability to combine two symbols to create a message, with a visual cue. Lucy also successfully categorized items (i.e., *cherries* in the *fruit* category) in three out of four trials. During the test, Lucy frequently pointed to the visuals provided to communicate messages; however, during the storytelling trials she verbalized concrete features of the story: *"flowers"* and *"dress"* when talking about a wedding. Additionally, Lucy often attempted to spell responses; however, she often only wrote a single word or phrase.

Feature Matching Assessment

Following these assessments, the SLP analyzed the results to create a list of iPad-based communication apps based on Lucy's strengths and needs – as well as her preferences. This process, known as feature matching, pairs an individual with an app or device tailored to their strengths and weaknesses, that best fits a person's current and future communicative needs (Gosnell et al., 2011). Feature matching is a critical aspect of AAC assessment given that there is a high rate of device abandonment (Johnson et al., 2006). In fact, "poor fit" of a device is considered a primary cause of AAC abandonment (Johnson et al., 2006, p. 93). Specifically, "poor fit" is described as:

1. "System not functionally used."
2. "System difficult to use."
3. "Mismatch between person and system" (p. 94).

In the case of Lucy, the SLP aimed to avoid abandonment by ensuring the features of an app matched Lucy's abilities and needs. To achieve this goal, the clinician considered the information from the assessments and identified a number of app features as important, as illustrated in Table 9.5.

Identification of Contextual Facilitators and Barriers

AAC facilitators are people, policies, attitudes, or environments that motivate and ease use for the AAC user (American Speech-Language-Hearing Association, 2020b). AAC barriers are personal or environmental factors that hinder

Table 9.5 Summary of Feature Matching Decisions

FEATURES	RATIONALE	
Hybrid Display	Visual Scene Display (VSD)	Traditional Grid
	• Used photographs in a sequential manner to tell stories	• Learned how to manage the Symbol Trails task on the CLQT (Helm-Estabrooks, 2001)
	• Pointed to visuals to communicate her intended message during the MCST-A (Garret & Lasker, 2007c)	• Read with fair accuracy (WAB-R) (Kertesz, 2006)
	• Navigated her device more readily with a navigation ring (within the VSD software), in observation	• Partially spelled words (WAB-R; MCST-A) (Kertesz, 2006; Garret & Lasker, 2007c)
	• During the interview with the SLP, Lucy used relevant images to expand upon her spoken expression	• Categorized vocabulary on MCST-A (Garret & Lasker, 2007c)
		• Navigated the stimulus book of the MCST-A (Garret & Lasker, 2007c) to answer questions
QWERTY keyboard with word prediction	• Lucy reported that she was comfortable using the iPhone keyboard to text and send messages on Facebook	
	• During the interview with the SLP, Lucy turned to the QWERTY keyboard to augment spoken expression	
	• Read with fair accuracy (WAB-R) (Kertesz, 2006)	
	• Partially spelled words (WAB-R, MCST-A) (Kertesz, 2006; Garret & Lasker, 2007c)	
Ability to import photographs	• Friends and family remain important to Lucy; using personal images may increase social closeness	
	• Photos offer communication partner support during interactions (Hux, 2010)	
	• Using personally relevant photos that Lucy can import may increase communicative success (Dietz et al., 2014)	
Quick phrases	• Accessible full messages that Lucy can use to talk about medical needs/aphasia if there is a communication breakdown	
	• On the CETI (Lomas et al., 1989), Lucy indicated she would like to quickly talk about her stroke/aphasia	
	• Describing things at length is difficult for Lucy; pre-stored "quick phrases" may alleviate stress and frustration when she is required to describe something at length	

AAC use. AAC should not be a burden to those using the technology; facilitators and barriers should constantly be evaluated to equip clients with the technology best suited for them. Table 9.6 summarizes Lucy's facilitators and barriers.

Treatment Plan

The AAC-focused part of the treatment included five phases: device introduction, app exploration, guided practice, independent monitoring, and

Table 9.6 AAC Facilitators and Barriers

Lucy's AAC Facilitators	Lucy's AAC Barriers
• Lucy's family is supportive	• Low confidence in her communicative capabilities
• Her rehab team is knowledgeable about AAC	• Right-sided weakness limits range of motion for AAC access
• Clear visual field	

generalization, adapted from two studies focused on AAC for people with aphasia (Dietz et al., 2018; Hough & Johnson, 2009). These phases are explained in Table 9.7. To advance to a new phase of treatment, Lucy needed to show competence (85% accuracy) in the preceding phase. A checklist was used to keep data for each phase of treatment.

During active treatment, Lucy was seen for two one-hour sessions, five or six days a week during her inpatient rehabilitation stay. Each phase of treatment lasted approximately two to three weeks. At the end of treatment, Lucy had attended a total of 24 sessions. Throughout treatment, the clinician intermittently described troubleshooting techniques and programming instruction so that Lucy and Jim would be better equipped for independent programming and use at home.

Follow-Up and Outcomes

Prior to discharge home for outpatient rehabilitation, the SLP re-administered the WAB-R (Kertesz, 2006), the CETI (Lomas et al., 1989), and the SAQOL-39 (Hilari et al., 2003) to assess changes in Lucy's aphasia severity, current communicative status, as well as quality of life. The clinician also informally interviewed Lucy and Jim. Specifically, she asked questions related to Lucy's original goal, communicating effectively with her two daughters and relaying her needs to medical professionals. Jim commented on her improvements in communicative confidence. Overall, both Lucy and Jim agreed that Lucy was a more effective communicator; however, she continued to struggle with repairing communication breakdowns. The SLP encouraged Jim to create artificial communication breakdowns at home to encourage Lucy to practice her repair strategies. The SLP recommended that Lucy continue to work with an outpatient SLP on expanding her communicative repertoire and employing breakdown repair strategies. Social isolation and withdrawal are common concerns for people with aphasia (Hilari & Northcott, 2017). To address these concerns, the SLP recommended a local aphasia support group to Lucy and Jim.

Discussion

Creating a positive relationship between person and device is necessary for AAC acceptance. To do this, the clinician should acknowledge and incorporate

Table 9.7 Summary of Treatment Phases

Phases of Treatment	Description of Phases	Supplemental/Traditional Treatment Activities
Phase 1: Device Introduction	• Device orientation (i.e., location of charging port, on/off button, volume button, etc.) • Lucy, Jim, and the clinician collaborated to program the device using important photographs and vocabulary relevant to Lucy's daily life • Device navigation (i.e., navigating and opening Tobii Dynavox Snap + Core First: https://us.tobiidynavox.com/pages/snap-corefirst)	• Communication partner training (CPT) to introduce ways Jim could help facilitate communication with Lucy (e.g., using gestures, pointing, giving key phrases) (Simmons-Mackie, 2018).
Phase 2: App Exploration	• Clinician reviewed features of app (i.e., grid display, visual scenes display, message window, etc.) • Lucy was given time to explore features of the app • Clinician instructed Lucy to navigate to different pages of the app • Jim observed these sessions	• The clinician began semantic feature analysis training (SFA) (Boyle, 2010) to remediate Lucy's word-retrieval difficulties. • Photos and symbols from Lucy's AAC device were used as stimuli
Phase 3: Guided Practice	• Clinician used app to retell Lucy's programmed narratives; Lucy then practiced these same stories • Clinician offered visual cues, verbal and tactile prompts as needed • Jim observed these sessions	• The Sentence Production Program for Aphasia (Helm-Estabrooks & Nicholas, 2000) was used with Lucy to increase syntactic complexity and fluency • Sentences were created using Lucy's own experiences, as well as daily tasks Lucy was expected to complete in inpatient rehabilitation
Phase 4: Independent Monitoring	• Lucy practiced with Jim while the clinician observed • Lucy was encouraged to exhaust all communication repair strategies prior to asking for assistance	• Above treatment tasks were continued with scaffolding to reduce cues as needed
Phase 5: Generalization	• Lucy and Jim were advised to practice these skills with other professionals on the rehab unit	• The Life Participation Approach to aphasia (LPAA) (Chapey et al., 2000) was used as a map to ensure the current AAC app continued to meet Lucy's needs • Upon discharge, Lucy's communication needs were expected to change based on her environment and communication partners

the individual's strengths as a communicator (Light & McNaughton, 2015). Similarly, ensuring that the AAC assessment is "person-centric" rather than "device-centric" may enhance the AAC user's experience with the technology (Baxter et al., 2012). Including the co-survivors and caregivers in the treatment and assessment process is imperative for successful AAC adoption (Light & McNaughton, 2015). In Lucy's case, this meant including Jim in treatment sessions, implementing communication partner training, and the involvement of other rehabilitation therapists. The dual approach to treatment, integrating both AAC and traditional restorative language therapy strategies and overlapping stimuli, resulted in a generalization of strategies–and likely increased Lucy's willingness to embrace AAC (Dietz et al., 2020).

Patient Perspectives

Lucy and Jim were hesitant about using AAC; Lucy "just wanted to talk again." However, after the AAC treatment, they both reported they have been pleased with the results. Their initial hesitations stemmed from their concerns that AAC might halt verbal expression. Jim reported that he was satisfied with the explicit instruction he received during communication partner training, as well as instructional support regarding app use. Lucy continues to make improvements and remains in outpatient speech-language therapy working on communication repair strategies and expanding verbal expression.

References

American Speech-Language-Hearing Association. (2020a). *Practice portal: Aphasia*. Retrieved March 24, 2020, from www.asha.org/Practice-Portal/Clinical-Topics/Aphasia/

American Speech-Language-Hearing Association. (2020b). *Practice portal: Augmentative and alternative communication*. Retrieved March 24, 2020, from www.asha.org/practice-portal/professional-issues/augmentative-and-alternative-communication/#collapse_1

Baxter, S., Enderby, P., Evans, P., & Judge, S. (2012). Barriers and facilitators to the use of high-technology augmentative and alternative communication devices: A systematic review and qualitative synthesis. *International Journal of Language & Communication Disorders, 47*(2), 115–129. doi:10.1111/j.1460-6984.2011.00090.x

Beukelman, D. R., Hux, K., Dietz, A., McKelvey, M., & Weissling, K. (2015). Using visual scene displays as communication support options for people with chronic, severe aphasia: A summary of AAC research and future research directions. *Augmentative and Alternative Communication, 31*(3), 234–245. doi:10.3109/07434618.2015.1052152

Binger, C., Ball, L., Dietz, A., Kent-Walsh, J., Lasker, J., Lund, S., . . . Quach, W. (2012). Personnel roles in the AAC assessment process. *Augmentative and Alternative Communication, 28*(4), 278–288. doi:10.3109/07434618.2012.716079

Boyle, M. (2010). Semantic feature analysis treatment for aphasic word retrieval impairments: What's in a name? *Topics in Stroke Rehabilitation, 17*(6), 411–422. doi:10.1310/tsr1706-411

Chapey, R., Duchan, J. F., Elman, R. J., Garcia, L. J., Kagan, A., Lyon, J. G., . . . Simmons Mackie, N. (2000). Life participation approach to aphasia: A statement of values for the future. *ASHA Leader, 5*(3), 4–6. https://doi.org/10.1044/leader.FTR.05032000.4

Dietz, A., Hux, K., McKelvey, M. L., Beukelman, D. R., & Weissling, K. (2009). Reading comprehension by people with chronic aphasia: A comparison of three levels of visuographic contextual support. *Aphasiology, 23*(7–8), 1053–1064. doi:10.1080/02687030802635832

Dietz, A., Vannest, J., Maloney, T., Altaye, M., Holland, S., & Szaflarski, J. P. (2018). The feasibility of improving discourse in people with aphasia through AAC: Clinical and functional MRI correlates. *Aphasiology, 32*(6), 693–719. doi:10.1080/02687038.2018. 1447641

Dietz, A., Wallace, S. E., & Weissling, K. (2020). Revisiting the role of augmentative and alternative communication in aphasia rehabilitation. *American Journal of Speech-Language Pathology*, 1–5. doi:10.1044/2019_AJSLP-19-00041

Dietz, A., Weissling, K., Griffith, J., McKelvey, M., & Macke, D. (2014). The impact of interface design during an initial high-technology AAC experience: A collective case study of people with aphasia. *Augmentative and Alternative Communication, 30*(4), 314–328. doi:10.3109/07434618.2014.966207

Garrett, K. L., Beukelman, D. R., & Low-Morrow, D. (1989). A comprehensive augmentative communication system for an adult with Broca's aphasia. *Augmentative and Alternative Communication, 5*(1), 55–61. https://doi.org/10.1080/07434618912331274976

Garret, K. L., & Lasker, J. (2007a). *AAC-aphasia categories of communicators checklist.* Retrieved on April 9, 2020, from https://cehs.unl.edu/aac/aphasia-assessment-materials/

Garret, K. L., & Lasker, J. (2007b). *Aphasia needs assessment.* Retrieved April 4, 2020, from https://cehs.unl.edu/aac/aphasia-assessment-materials/

Garret, K. L., & Lasker, J. (2007c). *The multimodal communication screening test for people with aphasia: Scoresheet and instructions.* Retrieved April 4, 2020, from https://cehs.unl.edu/ aac/aphasia-assessment-materials/

Garret, K. L., & Lasker, J. (2007d). *Scanning/visual field/print size/attention screening task.* Retrieved April 20, 2020, from https://cehs.unl.edu/aac/aphasia-assessment-materials/

Gosnell, J., Costello, J., & Shane, H. (2011). Using a clinical approach to answer "what communication apps should we use?" *Perspectives on Augmentative and Alternative Communication.* https://doi.org/10.1044/aac20.3.87

Helm-Estabrooks, N. (2001). *Cognitive linguistic quick test (CLQT): Examiner's manual.* The Psychological Corporation.

Helm-Estabrooks, N., & Nicholas, M. (2000). *Sentence production program for aphasia: Administration manual.* Pro-ed.

Hilari, K., Byng, S., Lamping, D. L., & Smith, S. C. (2003). Stroke and aphasia quality of life scale-39 (SAQOL-39): Evaluation of acceptability, reliability, and validity. *Stroke, 34*(8), 1944–1950. doi:10.1161/01.STR.0000081987.46660.ED

Hilari, K., & Northcott, S. (2017). "Struggling to stay connected": Comparing the social relationships of healthy older people and people with stroke and aphasia. *Aphasiology, 31*(6), 674–687. doi:10.1080/02687038.2016.1218436

Hough, M., & Johnson, R. K. (2009). Use of AAC to enhance linguistic communication skills in an adult with chronic severe aphasia. *Aphasiology, 23*(7–8), 965–976. doi:10.1080/02687030802698145

Hux, K., Buechter, M., Wallace, S., & Weissling, K. (2010). Using visual scene displays to create a shared communication space for a person with aphasia. *Aphasiology, 24*(5), 643–660. doi:10.1080/02687030902869299

Johnson, J. M., Inglebret, E., Jones, C., & Ray, J. (2006). Perspectives of speech language pathologists regarding success versus abandonment of AAC. *Augmentative and Alternative Communication, 22*(2), 85–99. doi:10.1080/07434610500483588

Kertesz, A. (2006). *Western aphasia battery-revised.* Psychological Corporation.

Light, J., & Mcnaughton, D. (2015). Designing AAC research and intervention to improve outcomes for individuals with complex communication needs. *Augmentative and Alternative Communication, 31*(2), 85–96. doi:10.3109/07434618.2015.1036458

Lomas, J., Pickard, L., Bester, S., Elbard, H., Finlayson, A., & Zoghaib, C. (1989). The communicative effectiveness index – development and psychometric evaluation of a functional communication measure for adult aphasia. *Journal of Speech and Hearing Disorders, 54*(1), 113–124. doi:10.1044/jshd.5401.113

McNaughton, D., & Light, J. (2013). The iPad and mobile technology revolution: Benefits and challenges for individuals who require augmentative and alternative communication. *Augmentative and Alternative Communication, 29*(2), 107–116. doi:10.3109/07434618.2013.784930

Purdy, M., & Van Dyke, J. A. (2011). Multimodal communication training in aphasia: A pilot study. *Journal of Medical Speech-Language Pathology, 19*(3), 45–53. PMID: 24558295; PMCID: PMC3927416.

Rose, M. L., Raymer, A. M., Lanyon, L. E., & Attard, M. C. (2013). A systematic review of gesture treatments for post-stroke aphasia. *Aphasiology: Gesture & Aphasia, 27*(9), 1090–1127. doi:10.1080/02687038.2013.805726

Rose, T. A., Worrall, L. E., Hickson, L. M., & Hoffmann, T. C. (2012). Guiding principles for printed education materials: Design preferences of people with aphasia. International *Journal of Speech-Language Pathology, 14*(1), 11–23. doi:10.3109/17549507.2011.631583

Simmons-Mackie, N. (2018). Communication partner training in aphasia: Reflections on communication accommodation theory. *Aphasiology, 32*(10), 1215–1224. doi:10.1080/0 2687038.2018.1428282

Taylor, S., Wallace, S. J., & Wallace, S. E. (2019). High-technology augmentative and alternative communication in poststroke aphasia: A review of the factors that contribute to successful augmentative and alternative communication use. *Perspectives of the ASHA Special Interest Groups, 4*, 1–10. doi:10.1044/2019_PERS-SIG2-2018-0016.

Wallace, S. E., Hux, K., & Beukelman, D. R. (2010). Navigation of a dynamic screen AAC interface by survivors of severe traumatic brain injury. *Augmentative and Alternative Communication, 26*(4), 242–254. doi:10.3109/07434618.2010.521895

Wallace, S. E., & Kayode, S. (2017). Effects of a semantic plus multimodal communication treatment for modality switching in severe aphasia. *Aphasiology, 31*(10), 1127–1142. doi: 10.1080/02687038.2016.1245403

Wallace, S. E., Purdy, M., & Skidmore, E. (2014). A multimodal communication program for aphasia during inpatient rehabilitation: A case study. *Neurorehabilitation, 35*(3), 615–625. https://doi.org/10.3233/NRE-141136

10 Supporting Communication in Traumatic Brain Injury using AAC

Lisa G. Bardach

Background

Survivors of traumatic brain injury (TBI) often experience significant communication challenges due to pervasive motor, linguistic, and cognitive deficits and may benefit from the implementation of AAC (Beukelman et al., 2007; Campbell et al., 2002; DeRuyter & Donoghue, 1989; Doyle & Fager, 2011; Fager et al., 2006; Wallace, 2010; Wallace et al., 2010). Because the cognitive and motor performance of a person with TBI changes over time, an appropriate long-term AAC system can be difficult to select (Fager & Beukelman, 2005; Light et al., 1988). AAC intervention in TBI requires special consideration due to the cognitive sequelae that often accompany the injury (e.g., Wallace, 2010).

People who rely on AAC typically communicate at significantly slower rates than individuals who use natural speech and can be 15 to 25 times slower at producing messages than natural speakers (Beukelman & Mirenda, 2013). Because of the slow pace, conversation partners may lose focus and interest in the conversation (Roark et al., 2011); for all involved, conversations may be shorter or less satisfying than those involving natural speech (Higginbotham & Wilkins, 1999). Lack of engagement can be a significant obstacle to successful conversation in AAC (Hoag et al., 2004). While the challenge of time and pace is not unique to survivors of TBI, characteristics such as cognitive rigidity, lack of flexibility, and distractibility can compound the slow rate of communication, especially if there is an unwillingness to adapt a message due to time constraints or listener interest.

The success of a communication interaction depends not only on the skills of the individual using AAC, but also on the skills of the communication partner (Kent-Walsh & McNaughton, 2005). The support of key communication partners may be pivotal in determining success with, or abandonment of, AAC (Johnson et al., 2006). For this reason, training of communication partners must include both instruction in device use and in strategies to support interaction, and the practice needed to support the person using AAC (Thiessen & Beukelman, 2013). Supplying a speech-generating device (SGD) and providing training in symbols and syntax are not adequate to support the development of conversational skills (Kraat, 1985). Partner support through scaffolding

DOI: 10.4324/9781003106739-10

within interactions may be critical to promote effective communication. Scaffolding may involve partners' use of linguistic, navigational, turn-taking, and rate enhancement supports. When appropriate training is provided, in addition to providing the supports above, communication partners help to ensure that aided communication modalities such as communication boards/books and SGDs are embedded effectively in communication opportunities. Finally, training of the individual using the SGD needs to be provided not only in clinical and home settings, but also in the community (e.g., see Light et al., 2019 and the case described by Lasker & Bedrosian, 2001).

Client/Case/Patient Information

Kay is a 54-year-old woman who sustained a severe TBI secondary to a motor vehicle accident when she was 18 years old, resulting in profound dysarthria and dysphonia. She had graduated from high school prior to the accident and following the accident she still demonstrated intact spelling, as is common for individuals with TBI functioning at level VI and higher on the Rancho Los Amigos Levels of Cognitive Functioning (Fried-Oken & Doyle, 1992; Fager et al., 2007) She has lived with her father in his home since the accident and is supported by two brothers, a sister, and various nieces and nephews. She is unable to perform activities of daily living (ADLs) independently and requires 24-hour nursing care. She uses a power wheelchair for mobility, which she controls with varying degrees of success using her right hand.

Initial AAC Assessment

Kay was evaluated for an SGD in April 2000, having been referred by staff at her sheltered workshop. At that time, her level of cognitive functioning (LOCF) was determined to be consistent with level VII (automatic, appropriate) on the Rancho Los Amigos Scale – Revised (RLAS-R) (Hagen, 2000; see www.neuroskills.com/education-and-resources/rancho-los-amigos-revised/). History obtained during that initial evaluation revealed that Kay previously had used a Canon Communicator (see https://roa.atdevicesforkids.org/product/cannon-communicator/), a small device accessed using direct selection, with text output on a hardcopy printout or on a visual display but with no speech output, as well as an Epson Speech Pac (www.old-computers.com/museum/computer.asp?st=1&c=143) also accessed directly and offering synthesized speech output. No information was available as to when those devices had been acquired or who had recommended them.

Fager et al. (2006) suggested that abandonment of technology often reflects the loss of facilitator support rather than a rejection of the technology. The Epson Speech Pac had reportedly broken several years before the evaluation and, when seen, Kay was communicating with questionable success using an alphabet board and mouthing words. She exhibited very slow and inaccurate athetoid movement with her right hand, the only extremity over which she had control. Use of a keyguard allowed for isolation of individual keys and facilitated functional albeit slow access via direct selection. Kay's history of SGD use with the Canon Communicator and the Epson Speech Pac suggested functional, if not intact, spelling. Trials with various SGDs revealed not only functional spelling but also functional grammar and syntax. Following comprehensive evaluation utilizing feature matching (Beukelman & Mirenda, 2013; Glennen, 1997; Lloyd et al., 1997; Shane & Costello, 1994), a Light Writer™ (https://en.wikipedia.org/wiki/Lightwriter; last edited May 14, 2002) was recommended. Observation of Kay's cognitive impulsivity and rigidity coupled with reports that the idea of an SGD had been raised previously and met with lukewarm interest resulted in recommendation of renting a Lightwriter for four weeks to ensure her interest and its suitability for functional use. Kay accessed the device through direct selection using a deep keyguard (see www.spectronics.com.au/product/21836). The Lightwriter was mounted on her wheelchair for appropriate positioning, and it incorporated a visual display and text-to-speech output. The rental was procured and utilized, and ultimately the Lightwriter was purchased.

Kay was able to communicate messages through spelling with some use of abbreviation-expansion techniques and encoded messages to access stored messages. Abbreviation-expansion involves programming a stored message by using key letters to abbreviate a longer utterance (similar to the use of abbreviation in text messages). When the letters are pressed in the correct sequence with a delimiter key (such as ESC) to indicate use of a stored message, the full message is then typed in the display. Encoded messages are stored messages that are retrieved by pressing a specific sequence of characters and buttons. When the correct sequence of buttons is pressed (e.g., memory key plus letter H for "I need help"), the message appears in the display (Table 10.1).

Due to Kay's short-term memory deficits, cheat sheets were provided outlining the process for storing new messages (Table 10.2). At the time, Kay had many suggestions for messages to be stored, and the content of messages revolved around communication in the sheltered workshop, social settings, and getting her needs and wants met. Light (1988) suggested four purposes that are fulfilled within communicative interactions: communication of needs/wants, information transfer, social closeness, and social etiquette. Kay's identification of specific messages she wished to store aligned closely with this model. Kay was last seen by SLP in November 2000 and was happily communicating with anyone who would take the time to listen.

Presenting Concerns

Kay was referred again for SGD reevaluation in June 2013 by her case manager. An initial interview with Kay, her family, and support personnel revealed that she was no longer using the Lightwriter. Barriers included poor intelligibility of the synthesized speech, limited visual display making it difficult to see long messages during composition, and lengthy time for composing spelled messages. They indicated a desire for more intelligible synthesized speech, a much

Table 10.1 Examples of Abbreviation-Expansion Technique and Encoded Messages

Abbreviation-Expansion Technique	
Selection	*Message Generated*
PP	*I need to use the bathroom*
PZ	*Let's order a pizza*
INK	*I need a kiss*
BFN	*Bye for now*
Encoded Messages	
MEM + C	*Can you please charge my LightWriter™?*
MEM + H	*I need help*

Table 10.2 Instructions for Storing Messages on the LightWriter SL35™

Storing a Message Using the Memory [MEM] Key

Think of the message to store and decide what letter it will be stored under (e.g.,
  H = I need help)
1. Press [MEM]
2. Press [MEM] again
3. Press the letter to store it under
4. Press Y for yes

Storing a Message Using Abbreviation-Expansion

Decide what letters to use for the expansion code (e.g., PP = I need to use the bathroom).
1. Type the letters for the expansion
2. Press =
3. Type the message to store
4. Press [MEM]
5. Press [MEM] again
6. Press +
7. Press Y

larger visual display, and the possibility of using updated technology such as text messaging for communication.

Clinical Findings

Communication during the assessment was largely accomplished using a static alphabet board in ABC layout. Kay was noted to have difficulty reaching some of the letters, and it was often unclear which letter she was pointing to. She was observed to attempt to say letters verbally, but due to her profound dysphonia and dysarthria, intelligibility was very low. A highly skilled or familiar listener (such as her father and sister) could understand some of these verbalizations in structured or predictable contexts. Regardless, Kay continued to attempt to communicate using her alphabet board and mouthing words, even though this was largely unsuccessful, supporting the observation by Fager et al. (2006) that individuals with severe dysarthria resulting from TBI may not be able to judge the ineffectiveness of their verbal communication attempts. It was also observed that for Kay, communication of specific content often appeared to be less important than face-to-face interaction with another human being. In other words, the need to have the attention of another human being focused directly on her may have been more gratifying than transferring information or getting her needs and wants met, and may indeed have met her need for social closeness. Kay was adept at and consistent with error identification. She had developed a gesture with her hand that she used consistently to signify that the listener had guessed the wrong letter or word. She was determined to communicate and persisted until her message was understood.

Evaluation again utilized the feature-matching approach (Shane & Costello, 1994) and was accomplished through observation and evaluation of performance on functional tasks. No spelling test was administered; rather, observation of successful communication of messages entirely using spelling revealed functional ability. Success in locating targets in a field of up to 42 items with text-only labels and no pictures revealed functional literacy at the word and phrase levels. Messages communicated through spelling revealed intact syntax complete with use of grammatical morphemes. A keyguard continued to be critical in facilitating physical access. Alternative access was introduced and explored, but Kay was adamant in demanding direct selection.

Additional important features identified included a dynamic display to facilitate the use of stored messages by providing visual navigation rather than relying on coded memory, word prediction to enhance communication rate, use of color to facilitate quick identification of function keys, and arrangement of the keyboard page in alphabetic rather than QWERTY layout (similar to her alphabet board). Kay was given the opportunity to try out these potentially beneficial features on trial SGDs so she could see how they might facilitate communication.

Kay tended to gravitate toward the use of spelling for communication in general, and she was resistant to displays that had only icons or icons plus text. Brown et al. (2015) found that individuals with TBI located target items most rapidly in displays where icons appeared without supporting text. However, they also noted that perhaps the greatest advantage for using text as a method of language representation may be transparency, at least for literate communication partners. It was determined that Kay's strong preference for text as her method of language representation should be respected. However, an AAC system was ultimately selected that would allow for the addition of symbols should Kay change her mind.

At initial evaluation in 2000, Kay was participating in a sheltered workshop three days a week, performing data entry tasks using a computer with a QWERTY keyboard. At the time of this reevaluation, she had not participated in the workshop for more than five years. Furthermore, her low-tech alphabet board was arranged in alphabetic order. Kay was observed using both layouts in typing for communication, and she stated a clear preference for the alphabetic layout. The NovaChat 10® (https://saltillo.com/products#nova-chat-10) with a 42-location keyguard was recommended. Since Kay continued to exhibit impulsive behavior and lack of flexibility, a rental was again recommended to ensure functional use and interest.

Table 10.3 outlines Kay's strengths and needs as identified through this assessment, guiding the process of feature matching to identify the optimal communication system for her.

Intervention

Kay presented as a very friendly and highly social individual with a close extended family. She stated a desire to maintain social connections with all her siblings but especially with her nieces, nephews, and their children. Family gatherings were frequently held at her father's home. She participated in social outings, including game nights, bowling, boccia ball, concerts, movies, and shopping on a regular basis.

System Set-Up

Based on the feature-matching process and the outcome of the trial period, the Nova Chat with 42-location keyguard and wheelchair mount were purchased for Kay, and the Nova Chat was mounted to her power wheelchair with the frame clamp from the previous SGD. It is critical that people who use AAC have access to communication at all times, regardless of their physical positioning, and an evaluation must explore all the contexts in which an individual may need to communicate. Low-tech methods of communication such as an alphabet board were insufficient for Kay's communication, so reliance on these modes for communication in situations where Kay was not in her chair (e.g., when she was in bed) was not acceptable. A second mount was purchased to allow the device to be mounted to her bedrail for access in bed.

Therapy Goals

Intervention took into account many aspects of Kay's personality, including her overall desire to socialize. Therapy focused on (a) identifying and categorizing stored messages; (b) using stored messages in functional ways (e.g., non-obligatory commenting, social interactions, getting attention); and (c) ways to enhance communication rate, especially with family and friends. For Kay to be an effective communicator, she required access to spelling for communication of novel messages, but she also needed to learn to exploit stored messages that might not reflect her exact words but that would express the same concept with

Table 10.3 Summary of Strengths and Needs Identified on Assessment

Domain	Strengths	Needs	Challenges
Linguistic	• Functional speller • Good use of syntax • Functional literacy	• Keyboard with message display • Auditory feedback to reduce errors	• Perseverates on spelling
Operational	• Navigates through various screens • Good concrete categorization skills • Uses function keys such as clear, backspace, delete word • Can use word prediction	• Store messages via category • Function keys on keyboard to refine message • Word prediction that learns new words	• Difficulty with physical access and isolating fingers • Too much navigation significantly increases time needed to generate message
Social	• Good sense of humor • Loves to interact with people • Participates in a variety of social outings	• Stored messages for quick social interaction • Ability to comment and share opinions quickly	• Has gotten used to being "talked over" • Will listen to conversation of others rather than trying to introduce new topic
Strategic	• Uses gesture to indicate when listener guessed wrong • Asks for changes to be made to SGD • Uses single letters and numbers instead of whole words (U, R, 2)	• Create cross-navigational options (e.g., can get to some categories from other categories instead of navigating back to home page) • Checkerboard pattern and use of color to facilitate visual identification of stored messages	• Loses out on multiple communication opportunities due to slow message formulation

much greater speed. Goals to improve her communication efficiency when using spelling included communicating key information in a small number of words and using word prediction effectively.

Enhancing Efficiency, Reducing Operational Demands

Unless an individual only requires access to a small number of messages in their SGD, it will be necessary to navigate through one or more screens to get to the desired message. Thus, the number of messages to be stored must be balanced with the navigation demands. Visual (e.g., color coding) and cognitive supports (e.g., organizational layout) can be critical for maximizing communication efficiency. While a particular message or taxonomic organizational structure may make sense to the SLP, or even to a family member, caregiver, or other communication partner, ultimately it is the individual using AAC who must locate the vocabulary during a communication exchange. Wallace et al. (2010) suggested that cognitive flexibility affects AAC system navigation. Because individuals with TBI often lack cognitive flexibility, it is critical that they participate actively in the determination of messages to be stored and the organizational structure under which they will be stored.

Customization of the Nova Chat occurred over many sessions, making sure that Kay was included in vocabulary selection and determining the organizational structure for pages with stored messages (see Figure 10.1). To facilitate motor planning and automaticity, a template was created for all pages (see Figure 10.2), including the spelling page, that placed function and navigation buttons in the same location on each page. To promote quick communication without the need for constant navigation, "yes" and "no" buttons that produced verbal but not written output were placed in the same location on all pages. Categories of stored messages were generated and revised over time and incorporated different communication needs (see the list of categories in Appendix 10.A).

Various strategies were used to facilitate Kay's efficiency with the keyboard and with locating and using stored messages. The keyboard was set to speak each key (including function keys) out loud, providing confirmation of letter or item selection while reducing the need to constantly shift visual attention from the keyboard itself to the message window. Colours were used to differentiate function buttons. Colours were also used on some of the stored messages to differentiate types of messages, for example, positive and negative items on the FEELINGS page (Figure 10.3), carrier phrases versus content words on the HOLIDAYS and TV pages (Figure 10.4). Items that may have initially been placed in one category were moved to a different category when the SLP noted that Kay consistently looked for those items in different locations.

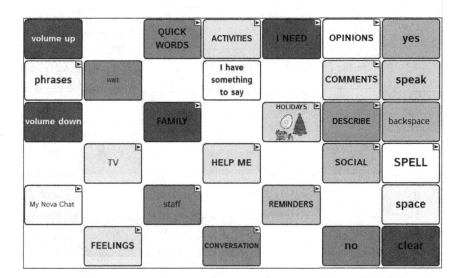

Figure 10.1 Organisational structure of home page

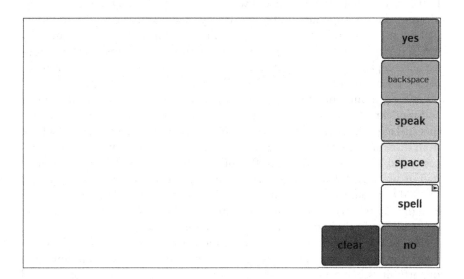

Figure 10.2 Template for page development

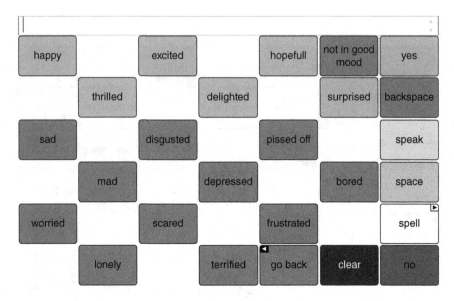

Figure 10.3 Colour coding for positive and negative messages (positive words are coded in light gray and negative words are coded in dark gray)

Supporting Communication Partners

Initial training with the system and with the concept of SGD use for communication was implemented with some family members and home staff. Home staff fluctuated significantly, and in spite of repeated invitations and requests by the SLP, training on Kay's communication with her SGD was not mandatory for any employees coming to her home. Kay's father agreed to make it mandatory for all home staff to put the SGD and mount on Kay's power wheelchair for a minimum of two hours daily. The SLP provided regular training and modeling to any home staff and family who were present during weekly speech-language therapy sessions and strongly encouraged input and feedback from those individuals regarding vocabulary, efficacy, and communication successes and breakdowns. As the SLP continued to solicit input from the regular staff, it was noted that those individuals began to demonstrate new interest in the SGD, encouraging Kay to use her SGD rather than her alphabet board and bringing up topics of conversation or activities that had been attended or were being planned to facilitate meaningful communication.

The SLP noted that most communication partners did not attend to Kay when she was composing a message. She observed multiple communication opportunities being lost because Kay's lengthy message composition resulted in many partners simply walking away. Settings on the keyboard page were adjusted to enhance attention, including activating the features of speaking

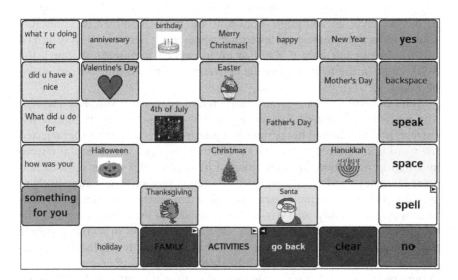

Figure 10.4 Carrier phrases + Content words

each word aloud (to keep partners' attention) and speaking each letter aloud (to confirm Kay's selection of the correct letter). The stored phrase *"I have something to say"* was added as a way for Kay to get attention, either prior to beginning her message or after completing it.

As noted by Fager et al. (2019), in an effort to decrease effort and/or increase the rate of communication, particularly in aided interactions involving spelling, conversation partners often provide spoken word choices to the person using the SGD during message composition, on the basis of letters already selected. This strategy can be disruptive and distracting, as the aided communicator shifts attention from message composition to the conversation partner to confirm or reject suggestions and it also risks shifting control of the conversation. However, when finely attuned and agreed between the conversation participants, this strategy can enhance conversational rate and reduce physical demands on the aided communicator (Roark et al., 2011; Fager et al., 2019). It requires the active attention of conversation partners during message composition and can exploit their familiarity with the aided communicator and the conversational context to generate better, more personal word prediction options than those generated solely using computational models. While there are emerging technological applications to support this strategy (see the SmartPredict app described by Fager et al., 2019; https://rerc-aac.psu.edu/development/d3-developing-a-smart-predictor-app-for-aac-conversation/), at the time of writing these options were still in development.

The SLP discussed with Kay the possible risks and benefits of allowing conversational partners to predict and provide physical assistance by directly typing any words correctly predicted into her message. It was agreed that allowing the partner to physically add single words into the message ensured that only Kay could produce the message in its entirety, reasserting her control. Kay agreed to this strategy, but only if Kay had given explicit permission to touch the SGD, either at the beginning of the conversation or each time a word was to be added.

Aides and staff were specifically instructed to guess what word Kay was typing, when they could do so with reasonable assumption that the guess was correct. If Kay indicated her partner had guessed correctly, the partner selected the word if it appeared in the SGD prediction, or typed letters until the word appeared in prediction and then selected it. Because the system software was set to learn new predictions, any word selected in prediction was more likely to appear again when the prefix was typed. Kay demonstrated significant fluctuation in physical ability on a day-to-day basis, in line with the observation by Fager et al. (2006), that during both acute and late stages of recovery, people with traumatic brain injuries present with a progression of changing needs rather than with a stable profile. On days when physical access was good, communication partners were encouraged to simply point out that the word was available in the prediction. On days when access was poor, partners were instructed to select the word from prediction if it was offered. While this form of operational co-construction carries some risks, exploration of strategies that work for a given individual with mutually agreed guidelines can provide new evidence for alternative intervention options. For Kay, having her communication partner physically select words from the prediction often resulted in effective communication of a message rather than abandonment of the communication attempt.

Intervention Outcomes

By involving Kay and her communication partners in the evaluation, an SGD was selected that Kay was motivated to use. Key intervention outcomes included the development of pages with stored messages that were meaningful to Kay and made navigational sense to her; use of a different form of operational co-construction that allowed her to continue to use spelling for communication but took into account the inconsistency of her physical access; involvement of communication partners in ongoing intervention to facilitate communication and carryover; and manipulation of settings on the SGD that facilitated interaction and partner involvement, such as stored messages for getting attention, having letters and function keys produce voice output to facilitate error recognition, and having words spoken aloud when typed to maintain a partner connection.

Further Update

In 2018, Kay was reassessed, in part due to concerns about increasing challenges in physical access, making use of the 42-location screen difficult, even with a keyguard (see Figure 10.5 for summary timeline). The outcome of that evaluation was a recommendation to purchase the Nova Chat 10.5™ with 20- and 25-location keyguards. This recommendation enabled Kay to continue to use the same familiar page set, transferring the vocabulary she had used for several years, but addressing the physical access challenges by significantly increasing the size of each target. Additionally, this choice reflected Kay's very strongly stated preference to avoid developing anything new; it exploited a degree of automaticity in message access, in that Kay already knew where many messages were stored.

In some ways, the new device places an increased cognitive demand in spelling: a page layout with a maximum of 25 keys means the alphabet must be split onto two pages to accommodate word prediction and function keys. However,

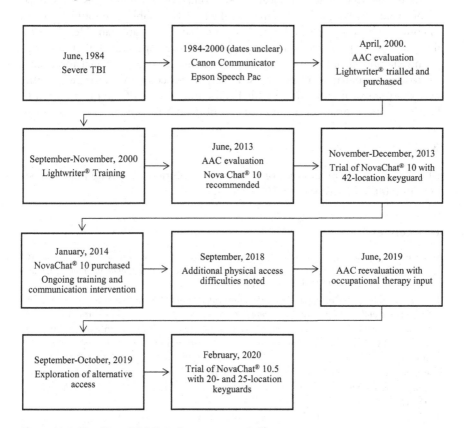

Figure 10.5 Timeline of AAC device recommendations

during six weeks of trial use, Kay demonstrated the ability to spell messages successfully using this system. At the end of the trial with the new Nova Chat, Kay wrote the following comment using the spelling pages: "I can't wait to get my new setup." There is no stronger rationale.

Conclusion

Kay's case illustrates several key points when considering AAC interventions for individuals with TBI. One is that AAC interventions for individuals with TBI are typically ongoing endeavours that may include multiple AAC systems over many years. The need for changing systems may be both patient- and technology-driven. In Kay's case, communication devices were abandoned for a significant amount of time prior to reevaluation and acquisition of new equipment. Fager and her colleagues (2006) concluded that when technology was abandoned, it usually reflected the loss of facilitator support, rather than a rejection of the technology itself. It is clear that ongoing partner training is a key pillar of intervention, especially for someone like Kay, vulnerable to multiple changes in communication partners due to frequent changes in care staff. Her case also illustrates the importance of focusing on individuals' language skills and recognizing the impact of impaired cognitive flexibility on organizational approaches to storing vocabulary and messages. Finally, Kay's constantly changing profile over the years of intervention highlights the importance of careful attention to linguistic, operational, social, and strategic domains in setting intervention goals.

Author's Note

Ms. Bardach is the owner of Communicating Solutions, a private practice specializing in the provision of AAC services.

References

Beukelman, D. R., Fager, S., Ball, L., & Dietz, A. (2007). AAC for adults with acquired neurological conditions: A review. *Augmentative and Alternative Communication, 23*, 230–242. doi:10.1080/07434610701553668

Beukelman, D. R., & Mirenda, P. (2013). *Augmentative and alternative communication: Supporting children and adults with complex communication needs* (4th ed.). Paul H. Brookes.

Brown, J., Thiessen, A., Beukelman, D., & Hux, K. (2015). Noun representation in AAC grid displays: Visual attention patterns of people with traumatic brain injury. *Augmentative and Alternative Communication, 31*, 15–26. doi:10.3109/07434618.2014.995224

Campbell, L., Balandin, S., & Togher, L. (2002). Augmentative and alternative communication use by people with traumatic brain injury: A review. *Advances in Speech Language Pathology, 4*, 89–94. doi:10.1080/14417040210001669311

DeRuyter, F., & Donoghue, K. (1989). Communication and traumatic brain injury: A case study. *Augmentative and Alternative Communication, 5*, 49–54. doi:10.1080/0743461891233 31274966

Doyle, M., & Fager, S. (2011). Traumatic brain injury and AAC: Supporting communication through recovery. *ASHA Leader, 16,* 2. https://doi.org/10.1044/leader.FTR8.16022011.np

Fager, S. K., & Beukelman, D. R. (2005). Individuals with traumatic brain injury. In D. Beukelman & P. Mirenda (Eds.), *Augmentative and alternative communication: Supporting children and adults with complex communication needs* (pp. 17–531). Paul H. Brookes.

Fager, S. K., Doyle, M., & Karantounis, R. (2007). Traumatic brain injury. In D. R. Beukelman, K. L. Garrett, & K. M. Yorkston (Eds.), *Augmentative communication strategies for adults with acute or chronic medical conditions* (pp. 131–162). Paul H. Brookes.

Fager, S. K., Fried-Oken, M., Jakobs, T., & Beukelman, D. R. (2019). New and emerging technologies for adults with complex communication needs and severe motor impairments: State of the science. *Augmentative and Alternative Communication, 35,* 13–25. doi:10.1080/07434618.2018.1556730

Fager, S. K., Hux, K., Beukelman, D., & Karantounis, R. (2006). Augmentative and alternative communication use and acceptance by adults with traumatic brain injury. *Augmentative and Alternative Communication, 22,* 37–47. doi:10.1080/07434610500243990

Fried-Oken, M., & Doyle, M. (1992). Language representation for the augmentative and alternative communication of adults with traumatic brain injury. *Journal of Head Trauma Rehabilitation, 7*(3), 59–69. doi:10.1097/00001199-199209000-00008

Glennen, S. (1997). Augmentative and alternative communication assessment strategies. In S. L. Glennen & D. DeCoste (Eds.), *The handbook of augmentative and alternative communication* (pp. 149–192). Singular Publishing Group, Inc.

Hagen, C. (2000, February). *Rancho-Los amigos levels of cognitive functioning-revised.* Presented at TBI Rehabilitation Managed Care Environment: An Interdisciplinary Approach to Rehabilitation. Continuing Education Programs of America.

Higginbotham, D. J., & Wilkins, D. P. (1999). Slipping through the time stream: Social issues of time and timing in augmented interactions. In D. Kovarsky, J. Duchan, & M. Maxwell (Eds.), *Constructing (in)competence: Disabling evaluations in clinical and social interactions* (pp. 49–82). Lawrence Erlbaum Associates.

Hoag, L. S. L. A., Bedrosian, J. L., McCoy, K. F., & Johnson, D. (2004). Trade-offs between informativeness and speed of message delivery in augmentative and alternative communication. *Journal of Speech, Language, and Hearing Research, 47,* 1270–1285. doi:10.1044/1092- 4388(2004/096)

Johnson, J. M., Inglebret, E., Jones, C., & Ray, J. (2006). Perspectives of speech language pathologists regarding success versus abandonment of AAC. *Augmentative and Alternative Communication, 22,* 85–99. doi:10.1080/07434610500483588

Kent-Walsh, J., & McNaughton, D. (2005). Communication partner instruction in AAC: Present practices and future directions. *Augmentative and Alternative Communication, 21,* 195–204. doi:10.1080/07434610400006646

Kraat, A. (1985). *Communication interaction between aided and natural speakers: A state of the art report.* Canadian Rehabilitation Council for the Disabled.

Lasker, J., & Bedrosian, J. (2001). Promoting acceptance of augmentative and alternative communication by adults with acquired communication disorders. *Augmentative and Alternative Communication, 17,* 141–153. doi:10.1080/aac.17.3.141.153

Light, J. (1988). Interaction involving individuals using augmentative and alternative communication systems: State of the art and future directions. *Augmentative and Alternative Communication, 4,* 66–82. doi:10.1080/07434618812331274657

Light, J., Beesley, M., & Collier, B. (1988). Transition through multiple augmentative and alternative communication systems: A three-year case study of a head injured adolescent.

Augmentative and Alternative Communication, 4, 2–14. https://doi.org/10.1080/07434618 812331274557

Light, J., McNaughton, D., Beukelman, D., Fager, S. K., Fried-Oken, M., Jakobs, T., . . . Jakobs, E. (2019). Challenges and opportunities in augmentative and alternative communication: Research and technology development to enhance communication and participation for individuals with complex communication needs, *Augmentative and Alternative Communication, 35*, 1–12. doi:10.1080/07434618.2018.1556732

Lloyd, L., Fuller, D. R., & Arvidson, H. (1997). Feature checklist. In L. Lloyd, D. R. Fuller, & H. Arvidson (Eds.), *Augmentative and alternative communication* (p. 494). Allyn & Bacon.

Roark, B., Fowler, A., Sproat, R., Gibbons, C., & Fried-Oken, M. (2011). Towards technology-assisted co-construction with communication partners. In *Proceedings of the second workshop on speech and language processing for assistive technologies* (pp. 22–31). Association for Computational Linguistics. https://pdfs.semanticscholar.org/942a/943ac4b46ec 6d5a5c3e988e3e9a87cbf1ae9.pdf

Shane, H., & Costello, J. (1994, November). *Augmentative communication assessment and the feature matching process.* Mini-seminar presented at the Annual Convention of the American Speech-Language-Hearing Association.

Thiessen, A., & Beukelman, D. (2013). Training communication partners of adults who rely on AAC: Co-construction of meaning. *Perspectives on Augmentative and Alternative Communication, 22*(1). doi:10.1044/aac22.1.16

Wallace, S. E. (2010). AAC use by people with TBI: Effects of cognitive impairment. *Perspectives on Augmentative and Alternative Communication, 19*(3). doi:10.1044/aac19.3.79

Wallace, S. E., Hux, K., & Beukelman, D. R. (2010). Navigation of a dynamic screen AAC interface by survivors of severe traumatic brain injury. *Augmentative and Alternative Communication, 26*, 242–254. doi:10.2109/07434618.2010.521895

Appendix 10.A

Categories for stored messages

QUICK WORDS
ACTIVITIES
I NEED
OPINIONS
FAMILY
HOLIDAYS
COMMENTS
DESCRIBE
SOCIAL
TV
HELP ME
STAFF
FEELINGS

11 ALS/MND and Voice Preservation Through Voice Banking, the BCH Message Banking Process, and Double Dipping

A Case Report

John Costello

Introduction

Amyotrophic lateral sclerosis (ALS), or motor neuron disease (MND) is a progressive and fatal disease with a worldwide annual incidence of 1.9 per 100,000 people (Arthur et al., 2016; Chiò et al., 2013). From the onset of symptoms, median survival is 3.5 years (Traynor & Hardiman, 1998). With no single test to confirm ALS, diagnosis can take up to 10–16 months from symptom onset (Richards et al., 2020).

Speech difficulties occur in 80% to 95% of people at some point during disease progression (Makkonen et al., 2018) and early introduction of a broad range of communication strategies is essential. Not all strategies may be needed, but individuals should be empowered with information to support their decision making, enabling a degree of control over their experience with the disease. Offering control through AAC options provides hope that individuals can maintain social connectedness and a sense of self, and this hope can be powerful in helping a person cope with living with ALS (Kim, 1998).

Historically, the introduction of AAC for people with ALS/MND has often been delayed until speech intelligibility begins to significantly impact communication, most often out of concern about overwhelming families and individuals with ALS with the looming loss of speech. Traditional guidelines reference metrics such as speech intelligibility decline to 90% and/or a speech rate of 125 words per minute (Ball et al., 2001, 2002, 2007, 2013; Doyle, 2001). More recently there is growing emphasis on referral for AAC evaluation at the point of diagnosis, to maximize opportunities to bank messages and voice prior to changes in speech (Cave & Bloch, 2021; Costello, 2000; Costello, 2015; Costello & Smith, 2021; Pattee, Plowman et al., 2018, 2019; Smith & Costello, 2021) Given that dissatisfaction with voice quality can increase the likelihood of rejecting an AAC device (Alper, 2017), there is strong motivation to support people who may rely on speech-generating devices (SGDs), to engage with intervention as soon as possible and before their vocal quality changes significantly.

DOI: 10.4324/9781003106739-11

Discussing the need for voice preservation is rarely easy. Initially, a person with ALS may want to recreate or save their voice but be unclear how that could be accomplished. Others may show interest in the process of preserving voice, but they and their loved ones may be emotionally paralyzed at the prospect of losing speech, and what they perceive as an inevitably daunting task to preserve it. Counseling and rapport building are the foundation for initiating the message banking and voice preservation process (see Costello & Smith, 2021).

The Boston Children's Hospital's (BCH's) Jay S. Fishman ALS Augmentative Communication Program has supported more than 700 people with ALS in the past six years. Most were referred early in their diagnosis, with a goal of maximizing voice preservation and exploiting the potential benefits of AAC solutions. Each patient has informed the development of a protocol for AAC assessment and intervention that now includes speech enhancement strategies, amplification, patient-designed low-tech tools, alternative access options, partner training, attention-getting tools, home automation, message banking, and selection of AAC technologies. The strategy that most patients have used, and that has been described as giving them hope and a sense of control, is the BCH Message Banking Process.

Message banking (Costello, 2000) supports people to record and store personally meaningful sounds, words, phrases, sentences, and stories over time, using their own natural voice and intonation, capturing their unique personality and identity. This approach has evolved into the BCH Message Banking Process (Costello & Smith, 2021), a dynamic and person-centered intervention with six values at its core: individual ownership and control, preservation of personal identity, collaborative focus on social networks, flexible to changing needs, unique and customized to the individual, and a foundation of hope and empowerment. Extensive resources outlining the BCH Message Banking Process, as well as assessment and intervention supports and relevant videos, are available at www.childrenshospital.org/programs/als-augmentative-communication-program/protocol-assessment-considerations/voice-preservation/bch-message-bankingtm-process.

Voice banking involves creating a synthetic approximation of a person's natural voice (Costello, 2016) for text-to-speech conversion. It involves recording between 50 and 2,000 or more scripted phrases, which are segmented to generate a unique phonetic database. These segments can be recombined to create novel utterances (Bunnell & Pennington, 2010). Using a personalized synthetic voice means that any message generated in text can be spoken. However, a synthetic voice cannot yet replicate the cadences of natural speech, the timing and intonation of utterances, and cannot reflect how a person uses tone of voice to convey meaning (Cave & Bloch, 2021). The phrases recorded for voice banking are not functional utterances from conversations; they are constructed to represent the phonetic database required to create a synthetic voice.

For persons with ALS, it is important that goals can be achieved with the least amount of effort, time, and energy investment (Jay S. Fishman

ALS Augmentative Communication Program, www.childrenshospital.org/ALSAugComm). The benefits of high-quality voice banking must be weighed against the effort required to generate the necessary volume of recordings. In double dipping, recorded messages originally collected through message banking, are repurposed to create a personal synthetic voice (i.e., combining voice and message banking, or 'double dipping'), eliminating the need to record pre-scripted messages. To yield a quality voice, at least 500 and preferably 750 or more banked messages of sufficient quality are required (Costello & Smith, 2021). This case report details the range of strategies implemented to support Andrew as he navigated changing speech skills over 18 months.

Case Report

Presenting Concerns

Andrew was a 46-year-old monolingual English-speaking, right-hand dominant man, married to Angela and father of three children: Andy (15 years), Lyn (12 years), and Sanders (9 years). He was a high school principal, had served on the city council, and had coached little league baseball and softball for five years.

At age 45, Andrew noted an unexplained change in right-hand strength, evidenced by difficulty using nail clippers to trim the fingernails of his left hand, slight muscle twitching in his right forearm, and occasionally painful cramps in his hand. He initially ignored these symptoms and attributed them to a back strain he had sustained at a little league baseball camp. Within a week, he noted twitching in his right thigh. He made an appointment to see a chiropractor about his back strain. Five weeks later, the evening before his appointment, Andrew noted slight twitching of his tongue while flossing his teeth. Using his smartphone, he video recorded this for the chiropractor. He also noted increased weakness in his right hand, finding that manipulating the floss was more awkward.

The chiropractor identified a potential spinal disk problem that might explain the right-hand weakness, although she also noted a slight wasting of muscle in the right hand compared to the left hand. On viewing the video of the tongue twitching, which she referred to as 'fasciculations', she recommended a neurosurgery consultation prior to any chiropractic intervention. Four weeks later, Andrew attended a neurosurgery appointment. He reported he had had an unexplained fall in the hallway at the high school. He felt as though he had tripped over his own foot, and his right foot did not automatically lift as he walked. Although he did not sustain any physical injury, his ego was bruised, as the hall was filled with students and faculty changing classes.

On reviewing an x-ray, the neurosurgeon reported a slightly bulging disk but cautioned that it was unclear the symptoms, including muscle fasciculations in both the right forearm and thigh, could be related to the disk damage. On examination, tongue fasciculations were not evident but the video was noted as unusual. The neurosurgeon recommended that a neurology colleague from the motor neuron clinic review findings and conduct a further examination, scheduled for four weeks later.

Andrew's wife Angela accompanied him to the neurology evaluation. On meeting the neurologist, Andrew immediately reported a new concern. Two days previously, he had coached softball and the next day he had chaired a four-hour meeting during which he needed to speak for extended periods of time. That afternoon, he announced the award nominations to the high school using the public address system. After completing the announcement, Andrew's assistant told him that his speech sounded slurred, as if he had consumed alcohol. Andrew also reported that his right hand had become weaker and that he experienced fasciculations on his right side regularly, even when in bed. Angela confirmed observing muscle twitching when Andrew was sleeping. She also recounted that when Andrew was helping with homework one evening after coaching, their daughter was delighted that she could say 'Pythagorean theory' quickly, but her father needed to say it in measured syllables. Andrew initially stated that he was simply being precise but on further reflection, realized it was a struggle to articulate the phrase. He could speak the phrase fluently during the examination, having had a low-key and leisurely morning involving very little talking.

The neurologist conducted a thorough exam, including a family history, a physical examination, cranial nerve exam, blood sample analysis, EMG (electromyogram), and a nerve conduction test. After the lengthy visit, the doctor reported that she strongly suspected a diagnosis of ALS/MND. She highlighted that ALS can mimic other neurological conditions and that diagnosis is difficult and confirmed only by ruling out other conditions. Although further tests were recommended, she believed ALS to be the most likely diagnosis.

She recommended Andrew meet with physical therapy due to his recent fall, as well as a counselor. She added that given the reported changes in speech, she was referring Andrew to speech-language pathology to explore options to assess speech, eating, and swallowing and to introduce information regarding strategies to support successful communication if speech became difficult. She highlighted that the goal was for Andrew to learn of many tools and strategies so he would be well informed, even though he might not need any of these strategies.

Andrew and Angela requested some time to process all the information but agreed they would follow up as suggested. Additional medical tests were ordered over the next three months. The diagnosis of ALS was confirmed nearly seven months after Andrew noted initial symptoms. He expressed frustration with the time taken to establish the diagnosis but indicated that he had suspected it would be confirmed. His own research revealed that diagnosis can take even longer, and many people are misdiagnosed before ALS/MND is confirmed (Paganoni, Macklin et al., 2014). He appreciated that his medical team had been proactive, making referrals for clinical services before a definitive diagnosis.

Clinical Findings

Andrew was seen for an AAC consultation following the referral by his neurologist, who wished for message banking and voice banking to be discussed. He had already been seen by a speech-language pathologist (SLP) to assess motor speech as well as eating and swallowing function. This first session lasted two hours. Andrew was accompanied by his wife. He and Angela reported they were interested in 'staying ahead of the curve', learning strategies for immediate use and taking action to have more control in the future.

Diagnostic Focus and Assessment

Andrew completed the ALS Functional Rating Scale – Revised (ALSFRS_R) (Cedarbaum et al., 1999). He scored 46/48, with slight changes in the use of his right hand when writing and in clarity of speech when fatigued. He completed the general short form of the Communication Participation Item Bank (Baylor et al., 2013). His responses revealed that his speech changes did not affect communication function with any communication partners. Reading the Rainbow passage (Fairbanks, 1960) at his usual pace, Andrew read 189 words per minute. Based on interview and observation, his speech course was categorized at Stage 2 in the Staging of Dysarthria (Hillel et al., 1989; Yorkston & Beukelman, 1999; Yorkston et al., 1993), with speech changes noted by others, especially during fatigue or stress, and some episodic changes noted in speaking rate, but no impact on communicative function.

Andrew was asked to detail his goals for the consultation. He did not know what to expect but had been told that with the diagnosis of ALS, he was at risk of losing the ability to speak. His physician had encouraged the referral, citing clinical support he could receive to save his voice for the future. Andrew added, "My voice is who I am. My children, my wife, my students, my colleagues, my athletes on the field – heck even my dog, they all know me as *this* voice. If it is gone, a piece of my identity is gone."

Intervention

Andrew was first counseled to preserve energy whenever speaking. His professional life and his extracurricula activities (e.g., coaching) relied heavily on speaking. The muscle groups used in speech production were described, highlighting the simultaneous engagement of muscles of respiration, phonation, articulation, and resonance. The potential to use a personal voice amplifier to minimize energy expenditure and delay the onset of fatigue when speaking was detailed. Andrew agreed to trial the amplifier during the clinic session. After only a few minutes, he stated that he could relax and speak with less effort. Angela added that he appeared visibly more relaxed with the amplifier. The benefits of minimizing motor effort and delaying the onset of fatigue were highlighted. Andrew readily agreed to acquire a personal voice amplifier and use it at work, while coaching, and during other extended episodes of speaking.

Andrew was next introduced to the concept of voice preservation. He was told that if ever he felt too fatigued to speak or felt his communication partners were not understanding him, many tools could support successful communication. The right communication tool would be determined by a thorough feature-matching assessment (Shane & Costello, 1994). Based on his needs, strengths, and skills, communication tools and strategies tailored to his communication and motor profile would be considered. He was encouraged to consider voice banking as well as following the BCH Message Banking process to create an 'insurance policy' that he would hopefully never need. The concept of double dipping was detailed. The option to embed both banked messages and a customized synthetic voice in an AAC device was described, emphasizing the importance of only considering options that would work across all technology platforms, to keep future choices open. Throughout the discussion, Andrew and Angela frequently paused to wipe away tears as they contemplated the possible loss of speech, but repeatedly stated that they wanted to continue. Andrew was reassured that he was preparing for the probability of loss of natural speech but there was also a possibility he would not need to use AAC. He stated, "This is one insurance policy I do not want to have to use," adding "I feel like I am taking back control at a time when control is being taken from me: it gives me a little bit of hope."

Andrew reported that his first goal was to complete voice banking, to 'check it off the list'. He added that he was very interested in the message banking process as it was important to him that his children and wife hear his authentic delivery of messages, and that his children must always hear how proud he is of them. Andrew also revealed that to entertain his children when they were young, and more recently as a way of lightheartedly annoying them, he spoke using a Donald Duck voice. He wanted to record some of his signature Donald Duck voice messages in case it became harder to produce that voice in the future. He added that he always wanted Angela to hear his love and gratitude. He disclosed that in early courtship, he and Angela had invented voices that they used with each other. "I want to be certain Angela always hears that voice; it is part of our connection." Andrew admitted that he did not know how many messages he would bank and was unclear he would have enough to double dip.

Voice Banking

After reviewing a variety of voice banking options, Andrew selected one that required him to record only 50 sentences. This process was completed in approximately 20 minutes. Upon completion, an autoresponse indicated that Andrew would receive a preview of the created voice within 36 hours. He expressed satisfaction that this was completed and would be available if ever needed.

The BCH Message Banking Process

Message banking requires access to a small, portable, and flexible system that supports high quality.wav file recording and Andrew was loaned a hand-held recorder that met specifications. Time was devoted to discussing technical operation and use, as well as potential messages, including those associated with Andrew (i.e., 'Andrew-isms') and messages regarding self-advocacy, terms of endearment, personal needs, and other categories. A handout with suggestions, as well as a web link to an extensive list of messages banked by other people with ALS, was reviewed (see www.childrenshospital.org/programs/als-augmentative-communication-program/protocol-assessment-considerations/voice-preservation/bch-message-bankingtm-process). Andrew was reminded to continue to record messages for as long as he wished, knowing that future circumstances and life experiences with ALS might reveal other important messages.

Andrew practiced recording messages, including *"Nice to see you," "This is going to be fun,"* and finally, in the deep voice he had invented when he and Angela were dating, *"I love you my boo-boo bear."* He was shown how to save the recordings to a computer and upload them to a free cloud-based site: Mymessagebanking.com (BCH-TobiiDynavox, 2021). This site offers the facility for autotranscription and allows messages to be categorized and saved and then downloaded to many different communication technologies from multiple companies. After listening to his recordings, Andrew was guided on how to hold the recorder to ensure best quality.

Angela asked how the recordings would be accessed and spoken if Andrew ever needed to use them, leading to a brief overview of AAC technologies ranging from smartphone-based apps accessed with a finger, to eye tracking access and high-tech devices. All the tools reviewed featured examples of embedded banked messages and custom voice. Web-based tutorials were identified that Andrew could review at his leisure (see range of resources at www.childrenshospital.org/programs/als-augmentative-communication-program/protocol-assessment-considerations/voice/bch-2). Finally, the potential to use banked messages to create a synthetic voice by double dipping was discussed. It was cautioned that this process requires a minimum of 750 quality messages but that the larger dataset would yield a higher quality voice than the one created with the process already completed.

After nearly two hours, Andrew stated, "We have covered a lot and I have my marching orders." He added that he felt hopeful and empowered to be doing something productive to address his disease. He agreed to continue to follow the message banking process and to email when he had uploaded several messages to the web account, so the clinic could remotely check quality and offer advice. Andrew and Angela requested a clinic visit within four months and indicated they wanted their eldest son to attend. They believed he would be fascinated by the technology and comforted to help his father.

Follow-up and Outcomes

First Follow-up Appointment

Andrew and Angela returned four months later accompanied by their eldest son, Andy. Andrew walked into the clinic carrying a walking cane. The family had discussed his diagnosis in detail with Andy and he was eager to help his father in any way possible.

Andrew's speech was noted to have a nasal quality with imprecise production in rapid speech. He indicated that he spoke with much more care and paced his speech. On the words per minute assessment, his rate was 141. He had acquired a voice amplifier and used it in meetings and during evening family gatherings. He noted he would not return to coaching as he was concerned it was too fatiguing and he feared being less effective. He reported more difficulty speaking in competing noise, even with the amplifier. From Andrew's reports and clinical observation, his speech was determined to be at early stage three of the Dysarthria Rating Scale (Yorkston & Beukelman, 1999), with reduction in intelligibility and rate, and changes to resonance that, with effort, Andrew could modify.

Andrew had experienced several falls due to foot drop on his right side, with some minor weakness in his left leg. Angela commented that she wished he would use his cane all the time as recommended by his physical therapist. Andrew responded that he often used it, but he felt confident in the narrow hallway of the clinic as he could 'cruise the wall'. He reported more difficulty using his right hand for writing, using a keyboard, or holding objects. He agreed to see the occupational therapist to explore alternative keyboard access and assistive technologies.

Andrew confirmed that within a day of the previous appointment, he had received a link with a preview of his custom synthetic voice. It had sounded better than expected but he had hoped it would be more natural. Andy agreed that it sounded ok but emotionless. Angela and Andrew both were glad to have it but also glad to be completing the message banking process. They wanted to double dip, as they feared he might need to use synthetic speech in the future. Andy added "As long as you don't sound like Darth Vader," causing Andrew to paraphrase "Andy, I am your father," while Andy smiled and rolled his eyes.

Andrew had banked 440 messages, which he had uploaded and transcribed on the cloud-based account. He had also created categories including advice to children, messages to Angela, Dad jokes, Donald Duck voice messages, terms of endearment, reflections on faith (with two complete prayers), sports talk, household chores/requests, and social greetings/statements. As counseled at previous visits and detailed on handouts, Andrew had banked starter phrases such as, "*Would you do me a favour and . . .*". These phrases allowed him to capture his audience with his own recorded voice and complete the message with synthetic speech. Overall, the quality of the recordings was good. Andrew was reminded to take care when pressing 'record', to avoid an audible click at the start of messages.

Andrew wanted to bank more messages and was glad his voice was still strong enough. He commented on messages that he would never previously have considered, such as requesting assistance to massage his legs. He could no longer cut his own food and knew he would continue to need to ask for help. "I just want my family to hear the appreciation in my voice when I ask them instead of a robotic synthetic voice." Andy interrupted and reminded him that he had recorded no messages for Barron, their dog. Andrew picked up the voice recorder and recorded multiple messages to Barron. Andy prompted him to record " '*Dad voice*' messages – you know when you try to get us all to the dinner table." Andy imitated several examples, resulting in laughter from the whole family. Andy then grabbed the voice recorder and recorded Andrew while he laughed, stating that it was important that he always had his 'dorky laugh'. When Andy left the office briefly, Angela commented, "With this awful disease everything makes you sad, but capturing messages and recordings has been surprisingly enjoyable. I think it's been really good for Andy to have a way to help his dad. It is really important to have family involved." Andrew added, "and in a weird way, it gives me hope for my future."

During the remainder of this visit, Andrew was introduced to low-tech backup communication strategies he might need if he ever felt too fatigued to speak clearly. He also asked about apps he could use on his smartphone, especially those that allowed him to incorporate his custom voice and messages. A range of apps was introduced. Andrew was worried about losing hand function and wanted to understand how he could access technology if speech and hand function were too difficult. It was suggested that his referral to explore alternative keyboard access could be expanded to reviewing alternative access options for AAC technology, including trackball, head mouse options, and eye gaze access to technology. A four-month follow-up appointment was scheduled, with the agreement that he could return sooner if there was need. It was determined that the ALS Functional Rating Scale and the Communication Participation Bank would be repeated at the start of the next visit.

Second Follow-Up Visit

Andrew returned for a follow-up visit within 10 weeks. He arrived with Angela and Andy, seated in a motorized scooter that he controlled with his left hand using a large, balled joystick. He was wearing the voice amplifier and his speech was notably dysarthric with pronounced perceptual features of hypernasality and spasticity. He was judged to be in the later stage three of the Dysarthria Rating Scale (Yorkston & Beukelman, 1999) moving toward stage four, in which natural speech may be supplemented with AAC. Once in the clinic room, Andrew put his smartphone on his lap. With the ring finger of his left hand, he activated a message he had prepared using a text to speech app: "*Thank you for seeing me sooner. As you can see, things have changed a lot. I have left my job. I fell a lot within a month after our last visit. I was fitted for a power wheelchair and until it is delivered, I use this scooter. I can't use my right hand at all now and the fingers on my left hand are hard to use. My speech has changed a lot, so I use this app for long messages. I continued with the message banking process, and I recorded almost four hundred more messages but then about six weeks ago my speech got much worse, so I stopped as I don't like the way I sound now. I want to start using my messages and also want to double dip to create a synthetic voice."*

At the start of the session, the ALSFRS-R (Cedarbaum et al., 1999) was completed by Angela as directed by Andrew. Results indicated a score of 19/48, revealing significant involvement of speech, upper limb, lower limb, and some involvement of respiratory function. The Communication Participation Bank (Baylor et al., 2013) and words per minute rating tasks were not completed based on the status report delivered by Andrew.

Andrew's uploaded banked messages were reviewed. Since his last visit, he had recorded many new messages focused on personal care and had created categories of messages related to wheelchair, personal care assistance, hygiene, and medical appointments. Using a text to speech app, Andrew typed, *"I am so glad we followed this process and kept recording. When we started, I never imagined I would need to ask my son to wipe my chin, but you can see that is one of my messages."* (The message *"Hey buddy, would you wipe my chin please. Thanks, champ."* was recorded with a clear sense of gratitude reflected in the intonation of the message.) Andy added "I am really glad I can still hear you call me champ." The banked messages were checked for quality. Minor editing was completed and then they were downloaded from the cloud service and submitted to a voice banking service to create a voice through double dipping.

Based on careful interprofessional assessment and clinical trials with AAC technologies conducted along with occupational therapy over the preceding two and a half months, Andrew had identified an eye tracking camera and AAC software program that offered a suite of options as the best match to his needs. Among the key features was the facility to integrate his banked messages and his double-dip voice into the system. He commented, "I may have to use technology, but my personality is going to be built into that technology with my banked messages and my custom voice." One day later, Andrew's custom synthetic voice was created and a link to preview it was emailed to him. Angela replied immediately that she and Andrew were very happy with the voice. They felt that it was a good sign that, when using the online preview, they produced the sentence *"Barron, do you want a treat,"* and the dog stood up and walked over to Andrew.

Andrew's AAC device was procured within two months and mounted on his power wheelchair, and he accessed it through eye tracking technology (see Figure 11.1 for summary timeline). A series of trainings was scheduled with the clinic. On a follow-up visit Angela stated, "ALS has taken so much, but because we were supported to be proactive, we did not lose Andrew's personality. We hear it every time he speaks a banked message. We even hear it in his custom synthetic voice." Andrew responded by typing with his eyes the novel message: *"All I can say to that is . . .".* He then accessed his banked messages to add *"I love you my boo-boo bear."*

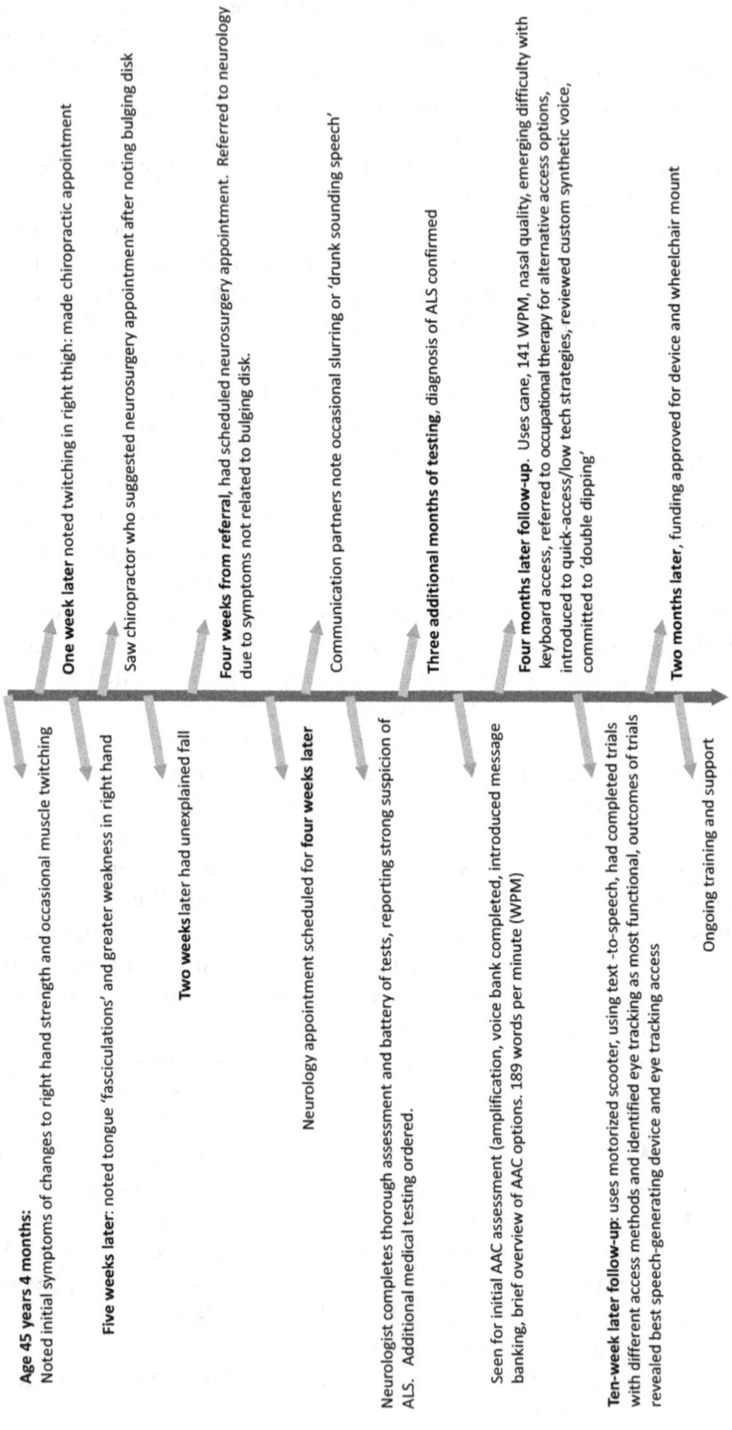

Age 45 years 4 months:
Noted initial symptoms of changes to right hand strength and occasional muscle twitching

Five weeks later: noted tongue 'fasciculations' and greater weakness in right hand

Two weeks later had unexplained fall

Neurology appointment scheduled for **four weeks later**

Neurologist completes thorough assessment and battery of tests, reporting strong suspicion of ALS. Additional medical testing ordered.

Seen for initial AAC assessment (amplification, voice bank completed, introduced message banking, brief overview of AAC options. 189 words per minute (WPM)

Ten-week later follow-up: uses motorized scooter, using text -to-speech, had completed trials with different access methods and identified eye tracking as most functional, outcomes of trials revealed best speech-generating device and eye tracking access

Ongoing training and support

One week later noted twitching in right thigh: made chiropractic appointment

Saw chiropractor who suggested neurosurgery appointment after noting bulging disk

Four weeks from referral, had scheduled neurosurgery appointment.   Referred to neurology due to symptoms not related to bulging disk.

Communication partners note occasional slurring or 'drunk sounding speech'

Three additional months of testing, diagnosis of ALS confirmed

Four months later follow-up.   Uses cane, 141 WPM, nasal quality, emerging difficulty with keyboard access, referred to occupational therapy for alternative access options, introduced to quick-access/low tech strategies, reviewed custom synthetic voice, committed to 'double dipping'

Two months later, funding approved for device and wheelchair mount

Figure 11.1 Timeline of intervention

Discussion and Conclusions

The option of message banking has been more widely considered for people with ALS/MND in the past decade. As people learn of successes achieved by others and as technology allows for creation of a custom voice, it is important to reassess the criteria for referral to consider AAC. Not all people embrace being proactive to the extent that Andrew and Angela did. The loss of natural speech is terrifying, and each person manages this news in their own way. Clinically, speech-language pathologists must guide people at risk of losing the ability to speak by providing all the relevant information. Given the data available and the variability of disease progression across individuals, it is important to provide that information in a manner that acknowledges partnership with the person with ALS, honoring their opinions while preparing a potentially unnecessary custom voice or a collection of banked messages.

References

Alper, M. (2017). *Giving voice: Mobile communication, disability, and inequity*. Massachusetts Institute of Technology.

Arthur, K. C., Calvo, A., Price, T. R., Geiger, J, Chiò, A., & Traynor, B. (2016). Projected increase in amyotrophic lateral sclerosis from 2015 to 2040. *Nature Communication, 11*(7), 12408. doi:10.1038/ncomms12408

Ball, L. J., Beukelman, D., & Bardach, L. (2007). Amyotrophic lateral sclerosis. In D. Beukelman, K. Garrett, & K. Yorkston (Eds.), *Augmentative communication strategies for adults with acute or chronic medical condition* (pp. 287–315). Brookes Publishing.

Ball, L. J., Beukelman, D., & Pattee, G. (2002). Timing of speech deterioration in people with amyotrophic lateral sclerosis. *Journal of Medical Speech Language Pathology, 10*(4), 231–235.

Ball, L. J., Nordness, A., & Beukelman, D. (2013). Individuals with acquired physical conditions. In D. Beukelman & J. Light (Eds.), *Augmentative and alternative communication: Supporting children and adults with complex communication needs* (pp. 519–552). Paul Brookes.

Ball, L. J., Willis, A., Beukelman, D., & Pattee, G. (2001). A protocol for identification of early bulbar signs in amyotrophic lateral sclerosis. *Journal of Neurological Sciences, 191,* 43–53. doi:10.1016/s0022-510x(01)00623-2

Baylor, C., Yorkston, K., Eadie, T., Jiseon, K., Hyewon, C., & Amtmann, D. (2013). The communicative participation item bank (CPIB): Item bank calibration and development of a disorder-generic short form. *Journal of Speech, Language, and Hearing Research, 56,* 1190–1208. doi:10.1044/1092-4388(2012/12-0140)

BCH-TobiiDynavox. (2021). *MyMessagebanking.com*. Retrieved June 30, 2021, 2021, from www.mymessagebanking.com

Bunnell, H. T., & Pennington, C. A. (2010). Computer synthesized speech technology: Tools for aiding impairment. In S. Stern & J. M. Hershey (Eds.), *Advances in computer speech synthesis and implications for assistive technology* (pp. 71–91). IGI Global.

Cave, R., & Bloch, S. (2021). Voice banking for people living with motor neurone disease: Views and expectations. *International Journal of Language and Communication Disorders, 56,* 116–129. doi:10.1111/1460-6984.12588

Cedarbaum, J. M., Stamber, N., Malta, E., Hilt, D., Thurmond, B., & Nakanishi, A. (1999). The ALSFRS-R: A revised ALS functional rating scale that incorporates assessments of respiratory function. *Journal of the Neurological Sciences, 169,* 13–21. doi:10.1016/s0022-510x(99)00210-5

Chiò, A., Logroscino, G., Traynor, B., Collins, J., Simeone, J., Goldstein, L., & White, L. (2013). Global epidemiology of amyotrophic lateral sclerosis: A systematic review of the published literature. *Neuroepidemiology, 41*(2), 118–130. doi:10.1159/000351153

Costello, J. (2000). AAC intervention in the intensive care unit: The children's hospital Boston model. *Augmentative and Alternative Communication, 16,* 137–153. doi:10.1080/07434610012331279004

Costello, J. (2015). *Jay S. Fishman ALS augmentative communication program | voice preservation.* Retrieved June 22, 2021, 2021, from www.childrenshospital.org/centers-and-services/programs/a-_-e/als-augmentative-communication-program/protocol-of-assessment-considerations/voice-preservation

Costello, J. (2016, December). *Message banking vs. Voice banking: A very successful proactive model for people with ALS/MND.* Presented at the14th Annual Allied Professionals Forum.

Costello, J., & Smith, M. (2021). The BCH message banking process, voice banking, and double-dipping. *Augmentative and Alternative Communication, 37,* 241–250. doi:10.1080/07434618.2021.2021554

Doyle, M., & Phillips, B. (2001). Trends in augmentative and alternative communication use by individuals with amyotrophic lateral sclerosis. *Augmentative and Alternative Communication, 17,* 167–178. doi:10.1080/aac.17.3.167.178

Fairbanks, G. (1960). *Voice and articulation drillbook.* Harper & Row.

Hillel, A. D., Miller, R. M., Yorkston, K., McDonald, E., Norris, F., & Konikow, N. (1989). Amyotrophic lateral sclerosis severity scale. *Neuroepidemiology, 8,* 142–150. doi:10.1159/000110176

Kim, T. (1998). Hope as a mode of coping in amyotrophic lateral sclerosis. *Journal of Neuroscience Nursing, 21,* 342–347. doi:10.1097/01376517-198912000-00003

Makkonen, T., Ruottinen, H., Puhto, R., Helminen, M., & Palmio, J. (2018). Speech deterioration in amyotrophic lateral sclerosis (ALS) after manifestation of bulbar symptoms. *International Journal of Language and Communication Disorders, 53,* 385–392. doi:10.1111/1460-6984.12357

Paganoni, S., Macklin, E., Lee, A., Murphy, A., Chang, J., Zipf, A., . . . Atassi, N. (2014). Diagnostic timelines and delays in diagnosing amyotrophic lateral sclerosis (ALS). *Amyotrophic Lateral Sclerosis Frontotemporal Degeneration, 15*(5–6), 453–456. doi:10.3109/21678421.2014.903974

Pattee, G. L., et al. (2018). Best practices protocol for the evaluation of bulbar dysfunction: Summary recommendations from the NEALS bulbar subcommittee symposium. *Amyotrophic Lateral Sclerosis Frontotemporal Degeneration, 19*(3–4): 311–312. doi:10.1080/21678421.2017.1404109

Pattee, G. L., et al. (2019). Provisional best practices guidelines for the evaluation of bulbar dysfunction in amyotrophic lateral sclerosis. *Muscle and Nerve, 59,* 531–536. doi:10.1002/mus.26408

Richards, D., Morren, J., & Pioro, E. (2020). Time to diagnosis and factors affecting diagnostic delay in amyotrophic lateral sclerosis. *Journal Neurological Science, 417,* 117054. doi:10.1016/j.jns.2020.117054

Shane, H. C., & Costello, J. (1994, November). *Augmentative communication assessment and the feature matching process.* Presented at the American Speech Language Hearing Association Conference.

Smith, M., & Costello, J. (2021). Clinical applications of speech synthesis. In M. Ball (Ed.), *Manual of clinical phonetics* (pp. 516–522). Routledge.

Traynor, B. J., & Hardiman, O. (1998). Motor neuron disease: Clinical features and management. *Clinical Medicine, 24*, 32–33.

Yamagishi, J., Veaux, C., & Renals, S. (2012). Speech synthesis technologies for individuals with vocal disabilities: Voice banking and reconstruction. *Acoustical Science and Technology, 33*, 1–5. doi:10.1250/AST.33.1

Yorkston, K. M., & Beukelman, D. (1999). Staging intervention in progressive dysarthria. *Perspectives on Neurophysiology and Neurogenic Speech and Language Disorders, 9*(4), 7–12. doi.org/10.1044/nnsld9.4

Yorkston, K. M., Strand, E., Miller, R., Hillel, A., & Smith, K. (1993). Speech deterioration in amyotrophic lateral sclerosis: Implications for the timing of intervention. *Journal of Medical Speech Language Pathology, 1*, 35–46.

Yorkston, K. M., et al. (2007). *Sentence intelligibility test, speech intelligibility test.* Madonna Rehabilitation Hospital.

12 Implementing AAC for a Person with Dementia

Adele May, Shakila Dada and Janice Murray

Introduction

AAC clinicians can anticipate seeing an increased referral of persons with dementia in the coming decades. This anticipation reflects a worldwide prevalence in which there are approximately 50 million people currently living with dementia and an exponential increase of 131.5 million is expected by 2050 (World Health Organization, 2017). Although age advancement is a key risk factor, developing dementia is certainly not an inevitable consequence of normal ageing (American Psychiatric Association [APA], 2013).

In the *Diagnostic and Statistical Manual of Mental Disorders (DSM-V)* (APA, 2013), dementia is classified as a major neurocognitive disorder. As such, it is distinguished by a progressive and irreversible neurodegeneration in one or more cognitive domains, (i.e., learning and memory, attention, language, executive functioning, visual perception, and social cognition). Notably, persons with dementia experience a significant decrease in cognitive functioning that gradually affects their independence in daily activities.

Dementia symptoms result from different underlying neuropathologies, reflected in differing profiles and subtypes of dementia. For instance, in Alzheimer's disease (the most common dementia subtype; DeTure & Dickson, 2019) neuritic plaques and neurofibrillary tangles in different cortical areas cause memory decline. A progressive narrowing of cerebral blood vessels may cause vascular dementia, and atrophy in the anterior temporal lobe results in semantic dementia, also referred to as semantic variant primary progressive aphasia (Gorno-Tempini et al., 2011). Other dementias include Lewy Body dementia and dementia associated with Parkinson disease. Dementia subtypes can often coexist, (e.g., Alzheimer's dementia cooccurring with vascular dementia) and accordingly present a unique set of symptoms. Despite the heterogeneity of symptomology, communication is invariably affected across the dementia subtypes, challenging both the person with dementia and their communication partners.

In persons with Alzheimer's dementia, for example, difficulties are often noted in auditory comprehension of complex language due to a decline

DOI: 10.4324/9781003106739-12

in attention and working memory. Word-retrieval difficulties may become evident by an over-reliance on nondescriptive words, (e.g., 'thing') which can be an early symptom of deteriorating memory (Bourgeois & Hickey, 2007). Likewise, persons with dementia may experience confusion with semantically related words (e.g., requesting a spoon instead of a fork), affecting meaning making and sense making for them and their conversational partners.

Over time, persons with dementia may withdraw from interaction altogether, and the resulting social isolation can affect valuable social relationships. With significant cognitive-communication decline, persons with severe dementia may appear nonverbal. Importantly, they may still desire to interact with others despite severe communication deterioration (Williams et al., 2003). Persons with dementia may be able to engage meaningfully with others by understanding the tone of voice and nonverbal communication (e.g., facial expressions) of their communication partners. Therefore, a combination of unaided and aided AAC systems, AAC techniques, and strategies can be tailored to support the changing communication needs of persons with dementia to maintain quality of life (Hickey & Bourgeois, 2018). Appendix 12.1 suggests some resources for persons living with dementia and their communication partners.

AAC interventions are not typically impairment focused, aiming to restore communication loss in persons with dementia. Rather, AAC interventions are aligned with social models of disability such as the International Classification of Functioning (ICF) (World Health Organization, 2001), which provides clinicians with a holistic framework in which to support persons with dementia to maintain independent functioning, engagement, and participation in daily activities. Within the ICF framework, AAC interventions focus on environmental factors (e.g., familiar communication partners) and personal factors (e.g., choices, preferences) to support communication participation and engagement in persons with dementia. To increase meaningful communication outcomes, a person-centred care approach is incorporated into AAC interventions to celebrate the life history and heritage of persons with dementia (Kitwood, 1997).

In a person-centred care approach, the personal values and uniqueness of the person with dementia is central to the assessment and development of intervention goals (Hickey et al., 2018). In clinical practice, this alignment can be achieved by involving the person with dementia and important stakeholders in their daily environment (e.g., family members, caregivers) in all phases of AAC assessment and intervention (McNaughton et al., 2019). However, although a degree of engagement is required of persons with dementia, the level of involvement is not imposed but rather is negotiated with them and supported in line with their capabilities and wishes.

In their routine clinical practice, busy clinicians need to engage in clinical decision making, but the evidence base supporting these decisions may be uncertain. Following the framework of evidence-based medicine (Sackett et al., 1996), Schlosser and Raghavendra (2004) emphasized the importance of evidence-based decision making in AAC defined as a triadic integration of (i) current empirical research, with (ii) the perspectives of relevant stakeholders, and (iii) clinical and educational expertise. These three elements are integrated and applied to the AAC assessment and intervention in the case discussed in this chapter.

This case report describes how AAC was implemented for a woman diagnosed with moderate Alzheimer's dementia. This chapter helps to answer two important questions often raised by clinicians: (i) What AAC strategies can be implemented for a person with dementia? and (ii) How do I apply a person-centred care approach within evidence-based practice in AAC interventions in dementia? The case report discussed in this chapter is structured according to the CARE guidelines of reporting case reports (Riley et al., 2017).

Presenting Concerns

Elizabeth is a South African woman, now aged in her eighties. She is an eldest child and has two siblings. The family had lived in difficult financial circumstances and as a result, Elizabeth hardly spoke of her early childhood years. Elizabeth married at a young age and had celebrated more than sixty years of marriage before her husband's recent passing. Elizabeth had invested much time in developing her career as a nursery schoolteacher. She established a child day-care facility and earned a strong reputation in the local community for developing excellent manners in the children in her care. Elizabeth was friendly and loved socializing with family and friends. She was known for hosting large dinner parties where everyone always felt welcome. Elizabeth was a talented guitar player and was a big fan of Elvis Presley. She took pride in her close-knit family and raised four children, one of whom, Rachel, lived in South Africa and the others in Australia. The family upheld Jewish customs and values, and these formed a significant part of their daily life.

In mid-2017, Elizabeth's daughter Rachel, who lives in the same neighbourhood, first noticed that her mother often repeated questions that had already been answered. Five months later, these lapses became more apparent as Elizabeth confused her daughters' names or used the phrase "what's it called" when she was unable to find a specific word. This pattern of forgetfulness was corroborated by Elizabeth's domestic helpers' observation that Elizabeth often misplaced her car keys and reading glasses or drove to the grocery store but could not recall the reason for the shopping trip. Initially, Rachel dismissed these concerns as normal signs of ageing, because her mother was approaching her eightieth birthday.

Elizabeth's behavioural symptoms became of increasing concern through the emergence of episodes of night wandering. Each day Elizabeth waited patiently at the front door of her home in expectation of her "boyfriend" arriving. She believed she was going on an ice-cream date, which had been a regular outing during their teenage years before the couple married. Elizabeth became highly distressed when she was told that this outing was not going to unfold. Worryingly, this daily occurrence continued for three months, prompting a visit to the family's physician. The presenting concerns raised red flags and initiated a specialist referral to a geriatrician. Elizabeth's independence in performing daily activities was impacted by a worsening of behavioural symptoms and a deterioration in physical endurance. Subsequently, just before Christmas in 2018, she moved to a care home within her local community. She appeared depressed and did not interact with other residents.

Clinical Findings

Early in 2019, at a visit to a geriatrician, Rachel was advised of the probability that Elizabeth presented with Alzheimer's disease. The geriatrician administered the Montreal Cognitive Assessment (MoCA) (Nasreddine et al., 2005) with Elizabeth. The probability of Alzheimer's disease was confirmed by a score of 14/30 on the MoCA, indicative of moderate dementia. Low dosage medication was prescribed for behavioural and depressive symptoms that Elizabeth had developed since moving into the care home. Further pharmacological interventions included adjustments to Elizabeth's diabetic medication, as she had recently experienced a loss in appetite and fluctuating blood glucose levels. There were no concerns about Elizabeth's hearing and vision. The geriatrician recommended nonpharmacological interventions in the form of music therapy. Speech-language therapy was recommended to encourage social interaction with others. These psychosocial interventions were part of a multidisciplinary management plan to increase Elizabeth's quality of life. A timeline of the relevant clinical assessment and interventions is shown in Table 12.1.

Diagnostic Focus and Assessment

A month following the referral to the geriatrician, Elizabeth was visited by the speech-language therapist at the care home. The clinician integrated research evidence with stakeholder perspectives and clinical expertise into her AAC decision making to support Elizabeth's present and future communication outcomes.

Table 12.1 Summary Timeline of Relevant Assessment and Intervention

Date	Relevant Assessment and Intervention	
Early in 2019	**Geriatrician consultation** *Cognitive Screening* • MoCA administered. • Probability of Alzheimer's disease indicated by MoCA score of 14/30 – moderate dementia	Recommended interventions *Pharmacological:* • Medication for behavioural and depressive symptoms • Diabetic medication adjusted *Psychosocial:* • Music therapy • Speech–language therapy
2019	**AAC assessment: Moderate dementia** *Research Evidence* Aim: To apply evidence-based decision making in AAC assessment and intervention	Strategy: • Consult reviews of current AAC research
	Multi-stakeholder perspectives Aim: To obtain opinions directly from Elizabeth	Strategy: Implement nonelectronic AAC to support interview • Visual support to support consent procedures • Talking Mats™ to support life story topic choice selection • Communication cards as visual reminders
	Aim: To obtain information from familiar conversational partners – Rachel	Strategy: informal interview Qualitative information • Family background, photographs
	– Nursing staff and music therapist perspectives	Strategy: • Walking interview with nurses • Informal conversation with music therapist
		Quantitative information • 18/30 on the DCDS: difficulties in comprehension, wording finding, and meaning

Clinical expertise
AAC customisation based on Elizabeth's:
Preferences
Self-selected topics
Current strengths
PC navigational skills

AAC system
• Personal computer (PC)
AAC symbols
• High context personal photographs
• Typed sentences in Arial font, size 14
AAC format:
• Life story sentences and personal photographs in Microsoft PowerPoint for reminiscence; enhanced with embedded music
Seating and positioning
• Seating changed for increased comfort
Vision
• Reading spectacles worn

Mid 2019 AAC Intervention: Moderate dementia
Goal: To increase communication participation with conversational partners
AAC system: Combined aided and unaided AAC
Elizabeth: Increase independence in using a life-story-based conversational support with communication partners
Conversational partner training:
• *Nurses:* To use life-story-based conversational support to initiate interactions with Elizabeth
• *Rachel:* To socially connect with Elizabeth by implementing AAC strategies in life story conversations

End 2019 AAC Intervention: Moderate–severe dementia
Goal: To maintain communication participation despite communication decline
AAC system: Combined aided (nonelectronic, paper-based) and unaided AAC

Early 2020 AAC Intervention: Severe dementia
Goal: To provide on-going conversation partner training and monitoring
AAC system: Unaided AAC to support care interactions with Elizabeth

Research Evidence

To familiarize herself with the most current research for supporting communication in persons with dementia, the clinician consulted two peer-reviewed scoping reviews, one of AAC interventions in persons with dementia (May et al., 2019) and a review of cognitive-communicative assessments in persons with dementia (Dooley & Walshe, 2019). To guide the development of a life-story-based conversational support, the clinician consulted an integrative review on life-story work by Doran et al. (2018).

Stakeholder Perspectives

The clinician consulted with various stakeholders to gain different perspectives on Elizabeth's communication participation in daily activities. These perspectives, in the form of interviews, were obtained directly from Elizabeth, Rachel, and other familiar conversational partners (nursing aids and the music therapist).

Elizabeth's Perspectives

Although the clinician attempted to introduce herself using a kind and friendly manner, Elizabeth appeared apprehensive about engaging with an unfamiliar individual. This reluctance may have been partly due to Elizabeth's not understanding the purpose of the clinician's visit, which was to establish rapport and obtain her consent to the AAC assessment and intervention procedures. Visual communication supports, in the form of pictures, were used to enhance Elizabeth's understanding of these procedures (see Figure 12.1). These visual supports appeared to make Elizabeth feel comfortable and she accordingly provided informed consent. Elizabeth seemed to experience each subsequent visit as a new encounter, due to her short-term memory decline. Consequently, the clinician used the visual communication support as an introductory procedure at each session.

During these sessions it was noticeable that Elizabeth struggled to initiate conversation and was unable to talk about her favourite topics (e.g., family). Furthermore, she was unable to maintain conversation on these topics even when they were initiated by the clinician. Conventional interview schedules were not applicable due to Elizabeth's auditory comprehension and verbal expression difficulties. Therefore, to facilitate these conversations, Talking Mats™ (Murphy et al., 2010), an interactive nonelectronic communication framework, was used (www.talkingmats.com/about-talking-mats-/#howitworks).

Using Talking Mats™ entailed Elizabeth placing three sets of Picture Communication Symbols™ (PCS) on a textured mat. First the conversational topic (e.g., music) was placed in the middle of the mat. Then Elizabeth placed conversational topic options (e.g., rock and roll music) according to a three-point

My name is (insert clinician's name). I am a speech therapist. I enjoy talking to people.

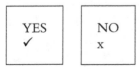

You can choose to talk to me.

YES ✓	NO x

If you do choose to talk to me, I will first do a short test on you. In the test, you will be asked some questions. For example, the date and time.

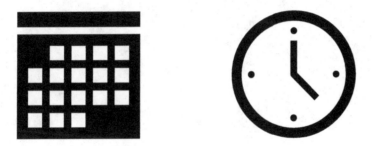

We could talk about your favourite photographs. You will choose the photographs from your family's photo albums. I will then put your photographs onto your computer. We can then talk about the photographs.

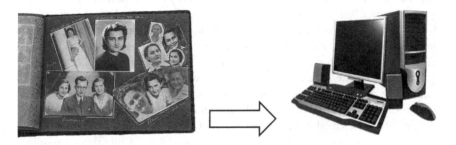

Figure 12.1 Visual supports for assessment procedures

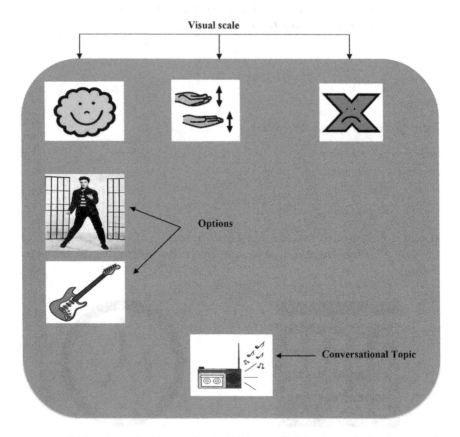

Figure 12.2 Nonelectronic aid example of a Talking Mat™ (Murphy et al., 2010) used with Elizabeth

visual analogue scale at the top of the mat to indicate her feelings about each option (see Figure 12.2). This structure aligned well with a person–centred care approach, as Elizabeth independently participated in decision making to select conversational topic options she preferred to be included in the life-story-based conversational support (i.e., Jewish family traditions, music). Accordingly, being able to chat about her preferred conversational topics was included as one of her initial communication goals.

Throughout the assessment, the clinician was mindful of Elizabeth's physical endurance and fatigue. Consideration was given to keeping conversations no longer than 30 minutes. Additionally, the clinician displayed picture communication cards as a visual reminder for Elizabeth that she had an option to take a break or stop at any point if required (see Figure 12.3). While these assessment sessions with Elizabeth were productive, challenges arose. On some days, Elizabeth did not feel well or was unavailable due to unexpected doctors' visits. Since

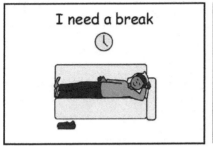

Figure 12.3 Examples of visual reminders during interviews with Elizabeth

these disruptions are expected when working with older clients and in particular, persons with dementia, the clinician rescheduled her visits accordingly.

Naturalistic observations were also performed to obtain insights into Elizabeth's communication in daily activities with different conversational partners at the care home. For instance, observations during group music therapy revealed that Elizabeth thoroughly enjoyed music in general. This was evident in her clapping her hands and humming along, even though she was unable to recall song lyrics. During observations of Elizabeth's afternoon routine, it was noted that she enjoyed playing memory games on her personal computer in her private room. A strength was observed in her basic computer navigational skills. Although Elizabeth had functional vision, she was observed to wear her prescription glasses to enhance the visual clarity of computer content.

Observations of Rachel and Elizabeth's natural interaction while reminiscing over general family photographs highlighted important qualitative baseline information. Rachel was unsure of how to support Elizabeth's communication, which caused notable tension in the dyad. Accordingly, Rachel identified that her communication goal was to learn strategies to connect with her mother again. Field notes were written after all naturalistic observations and were later used as complementary information for AAC intervention planning.

Rachel's Perspectives

Rachel's perspectives provided qualitative information about the family's Jewish traditions and family life. These perspectives embellished what was known about some of Elizabeth's selected topics. An informal interview schedule was compiled by the clinician to guide the interview with Rachel (see Figure 12.4). Additionally, Rachel provided family photographs, which were used to personalise Elizabeth's AAC intervention. Furthermore, Rachel self-administered the Dementia Communication Difficulties Scale (DCDS) (Murphy et al., 2013) to rate the frequency of Elizabeth's communication difficulties on a five-point scale. This provided the clinician with quantitative assessment information to

	Music Therapist	*Nurse 1*	*Nurse 2*	*Rachel*
What does Elizabeth enjoying talking about?				
Can you name some of her personal preferences?				
Which time of day is she most alert and willing to talk/interact with others?				
What other information would you like to share about Elizabeth?				

Figure 12.4 Capturing stakeholder's perspectives on Elizabeth's communication (Elizabeth's familiar conversational partners)

gain a holistic understanding of Elizabeth's communication difficulties (www. talkingmats.com/dementia-communication-difficulties-scale/). The results and interpretation of this assessment information are summarised in Table 12.1

Other Familiar Conversational Partners

The perspectives of nursing staff were obtained by adapting the format of the interviews to fit their busy schedules. This entailed 'walking and talking' while nurses continued their routine tasks. Nurses indicated that they did not know Elizabeth personally and would benefit from having more personalised conversational topics for interactions with her. By not imposing the need for traditional sit-down interviews, the clinician showed respect for nursing staff's time. Consequently, trust and rapport were established, which contributed to building a clinical relationship with nursing staff. Last, information from the resident music therapist confirmed Elizabeth's enjoyment of rock and roll music and specific song suggestions were recommended for inclusion into the AAC intervention.

Clinical Expertise

There was an opportunity for the clinician to re-administer the MoCA (Nasreddine et al., 2005) as it had initially been administered more than a year previously. Elizabeth scored 12/30 on the MoCA indicating that dementia symptoms were still within the moderate severity range.

Evaluation of All the Assessment Information to Inform Intervention Planning

Elizabeth's diagnostic AAC assessment and intervention planning was an iterative rather than a linear process. Clinical reflection was pivotal throughout. The clinician engaged in self-reflection through written reflections in a journal. This practice provided a channel for the clinician to evaluate some of her own assumptions in relation to cultural differences, and persons with dementia (Mahendra et al., 2013).

Overall, the AAC intervention was tailored to Elizabeth's communication goals, strengths, and personal preferences. The AAC intervention comprised a personalised story embedded within a life-story framework using Elizabeth's personal computer. The life-story framework included a story title based on each of Elizabeth's self-selected topics, with four to five short and simple sentences. These sentences highlighted happy moments, milestones, or memorable events in Elizabeth's life and were associated with a highly salient, context-relevant photograph (see Figure 12.5). Elizabeth's photographs were scanned onto her personal computer. The photographs were imported into Microsoft PowerPoint as the programme in which life-story slides were created. Preferred music was then embedded into selected slides to support the personalised content and enhance enjoyment. Together with the use of scaffolding strategies by a conversational partner, the life-story-based conversational support assisted Elizabeth to reminisce about personally meaningful topics.

My name is Elizabeth and I am Jewish.

Insert Elizabeth's
photograph

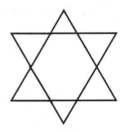

I love going to the synagogue.

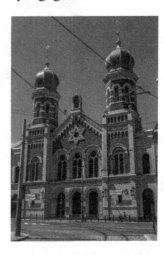

Figure 12.5 "My Jewish Life" (an example of part of Elizabeth's life story) *(Continued)*

Source: "Great Synagogue In Plzen" Image under Public Domain license. Copyright of George Hadan.

Every Friday night we celebrate Shabbat.

Monday	Tuesday	Wednesday	Thursday	Friday

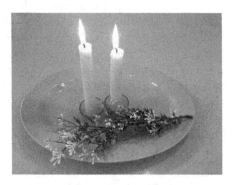

We dip apple slices in honey to celebrate Rosh Hashanah.

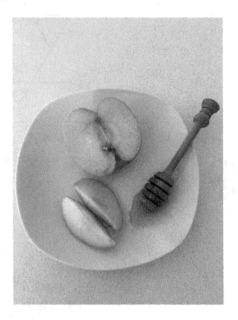

Figure 12.5 (Continued)

The clinician invited Rachel to view the preliminary content of the planned life-story-based conversational support. Additionally, the clinician trialled the conversational support with Elizabeth. This created an opportunity for the clinician to make adjustments based on Rachel and Elizabeth's preferences and feedback. Elizabeth was comfortably able to read the life story sentences, typed in Arial font size 18, on the computer screen with her prescription spectacles. Music was played through the computers' in-built speakers and the volume was adjusted to suit Elizabeth's hearing comfort. While using her personal computer, a regular seat was substituted for a wheelchair seat, as Elizabeth felt it offered greater physical comfort. Based on feedback from Elizabeth, no further adjustments were required, and the life-story-based conversational support was ready to be implemented with her.

AAC Intervention and Therapeutic Focus

The overall aim of introducing AAC with Elizabeth was to support her communication participation and engagement with her conversational partners. Initially, this was achieved by training her familiar conversational partners to implement AAC scaffolding options to increase turn taking and engagement within life-story conversations on her personal computer. The clinician implemented the AAC strategies independently with Elizabeth in two sessions, each approximately 25 minutes in duration, conducted over two weeks. With Elizabeth's consent, the sessions were video recorded for the purpose of modelling the use of AAC strategies as a practical training component for her familiar conversational partners.

Although Elizabeth was able to read the life-story sentences independently, she preferred to listen to the sentences being read by the clinician. To support Elizabeth's auditory comprehension of the sentences, the clinician provided AAC scaffolding by pointing to the photographs on the computer screen while simultaneously verbalising the sentences (Dada et al., 2019). Additionally, the clinician made comments on the photographs, supplemented these comments with gestures (e.g., "that is a *big* bow-tie"), and waited for Elizabeth to respond. Elizabeth used one form of interaction response, or a combination of verbal comments, communicative vocalisations (e.g., "uh-huh"), gestures (e.g., head nodding 'yes' in agreement), or pointing to family members she had recognised in the photographs. In other words, the use of AAC scaffolding supported Elizabeth to use multimodal interaction to increase her turn taking, but also to participate in an interaction with a conversational partner.

Immediately following the two sessions with Elizabeth, training sessions with nursing staff and Rachel occurred weekly, for 45 minutes over four weeks. At the training sessions, the clinician provided practical demonstrations of AAC scaffolding strategies. Additionally, the video-recorded sessions were used to demonstrate how the life-story conversational support should be implemented with Elizabeth.

The conversational partner training also highlighted how using Elizabeth's name during interaction and offering her choices of life story topics enhanced the person-centredness of the AAC intervention (www.alzheimers.org.uk/about-dementia/treatments/person-centred-care). Verbal feedback from nursing staff indicated that they immediately felt more confident to implement the

AAC strategies with Elizabeth. This further increased their willingness to initiate interaction with Elizabeth.

Follow-up and Outcomes

Two weeks post training, the clinician began weekly observations over a period of four weeks to observe the nursing staff's implementation of the AAC strategies with Elizabeth. They verbally reported that Elizabeth still enjoyed the life-story-based conversational support. No further adjustments were made. The clinician observed a follow-up session of Rachel and Elizabeth reminiscing together, using the conversational support as a scaffold. Enjoyment was noted by mutual smiles and laughter, taken as indicative of positive engagement outcomes. As such, the outcomes of the AAC intervention appeared to offer a qualitative benefit of social connection between Elizabeth and Rachel.

Six months later, Elizabeth's condition had deteriorated further, and she was no longer using her life-story-based conversational support. Nursing staff reported that Elizabeth was not eating and was unable to indicate her daily meal choices. The clinician utilised a simple nonelectronic communication board that included pictures of Elizabeth's meal options and yes/no response options. Nurses were shown how to supplement yes/no options with head nods to support Elizabeth in participating in making choices about her meal preferences. As Elizabeth's receptive and expressive language declined further, the clinician continued to train nursing staff to implement unaided AAC in the form of gestures and facial expressions to support caregiving interactions with Elizabeth.

Discussion

This case report described how AAC was implemented for a person with dementia by using various AAC systems while simultaneously applying a person-centred care approach within evidence-based practice. Accordingly, the two questions posed at the outset of this chapter were addressed as follows. In relation to specific AAC tools and strategies, a combination of aided and unaided AAC systems, techniques, and strategies were adapted to support Elizabeth's changing communication needs. Initially, in the moderate stage of dementia, the AAC intervention used a life-story framework delivered via a personal computer to support Elizabeth's communication participation and social relationships. Although Elizabeth's personal computer was invaluable in embedding personalised photos and music for supporting life-story content, careful consideration should be given to its possible limitations. These include, for example, the availability of electronic devices and the ability of the person with dementia to learn new computer-based navigational skills. Nonelectronic, aided AAC in the format of a communication board supported meal choice making. Gradually, as dementia severity advanced, unaided AAC (e.g., gestures, facial expressions) were introduced as the primary forms of meaningful communication interaction. A person-centred care approach was integrated into this AAC intervention by supporting Elizabeth's independence in decision making and using personally meaningful conversational topics. Ultimately, the implementation of AAC systems for persons with dementia is flexible and should be tailored to suit the communication goals and strengths of the individual client.

Outcome attainment was evaluated through a combination of direct observation and discussion with key stakeholders. One outcome of the overall intervention was an increase in Elizabeth's participation and turn taking in conversations, as her opportunities for supported interaction increased. In this regard, conversational partner training was an effective environmental strategy, as the nurses and care staff self-reported increased confidence in initiating interactions with Elizabeth and they were observed to engage in more frequent and longer interactions. Conversational partner training also ensured that the AAC intervention was implemented by different conversational partners, aligning with the ICF (WHO, 2001) focus on both internal and external factors in planning interventions.

Many persons with dementia can use language and, therefore, clinicians may not routinely consider AAC as a form of intervention for persons with dementia. However, Elizabeth's case illustrates how AAC scaffolding strategies can offer vital compensatory support for auditory comprehension and interaction in a person with dementia. AAC can be an accessible and valuable addition to other forms of intervention. Designing and delivering the AAC intervention described here may be perceived as overly time consuming for busy clinicians. However, clinicians may find that they apply many of the strategies described in this case report as part of their own routine clinical practice, without recognising them as AAC strategies. The description provided here is intended to support clinicians to adapt AAC implementation for persons with dementia in their respective clinical settings. Given the benefit of meaningful communication and human communication, the case for investing clinical effort in designing AAC interventions is persuasive. Furthermore, although applied specifically to a person with dementia in this case report, the AAC systems and scaffolding strategies detailed can be generalised to adults with other neurocognitive disorders.

Finally, reflective practice is one tool by which clinicians can strengthen their critical reflection skills and develop awareness of how to respond empathetically and respectfully to families — especially those whose culture is different to that of the clinician. These communication skills are essential for building effective clinical relationships with persons with dementia and with all other important stakeholders.

Useful Resources

Alzheimer's Society: www.alzheimers.org.uk/about-dementia/treatments/person-centred-care
Deep The UK Network of Dementia Voices: www.dementiavoices.org.uk/about-deep/
MoCA Cognition: www.mocatsajest.org/about/

National Institute for Health and Care Excellence: www.nice.org.uk/guidance/ng97/
chapter/Person-centred-care
TalkingMats: www.talkingmats.com/communicating-with-late-stage-dementia/
TalkingMats: www.talkingmats.com/dementia-communication-difficulties-scale/
World Health Organization: www.who.int/news-room/facts-in-pictures/detail/dementia

References

American Psychiatric Association. (2013). Neurocognitive disorders. In *Diagnostic and statistical manual of mental disorders* (5th ed.). Author. doi:10.1176/appi.books.9780890425596.dsm17

Bourgeois, M. S., & Hickey, E. M. (2007). Dementia. In D. Beukleman, K. L. Garret, & K. M Yorkston (Eds.), *Augmentative communication strategies for adults with acute and chronic medical conditions* (pp. 243–286). Paul H. Brookes Publishing Co.

Dada, S., Stockley, N., Wallace, S. E., & Koul, R. (2019). The effect of augmented input on the auditory comprehension of narratives for people with aphasia: A pilot investigation. *Augmentative and Alternative Communication, 35*(2), 148–155. doi:10.1080/07434618.2019.1576766

DeTure, M. A., & Dickson, D. W. (2019). The neuropathological diagnosis of Alzheimer's disease. *Molecular Neurodegeneration, 14*(1), 1–18. doi:10.1186/s13024-019-0333-5

Dooley, S., & Walshe, M. (2019). Assessing cognitive communication skills in dementia: A scoping review. *International Journal of Language and Communication Disorders, 54*(5), 729–741. doi:10.1111/1460-6984.12485

Doran, C., Noonan, M., & Doody, O. (2018). Life-story work in long-term care facilities for older people: An integrative review. *Journal of Clinical Nursing, 28*(7–8), 1070–1084. doi:10.1111.jocn.14718

Gorno-Tempini, M. L., Hillis, A. E., Weintraub, S., Kertesz, A., Mendez, M., Cappa, S. F., . . . Grossman, M. (2011). Classification of primary progressive aphasia and its variants. *Neurology, 76*(11), 1006–1014. doi:10.1212/WNL.0b013e31821103e6

Hickey, E. M., & Bourgeois, M. S. (2018). Cognitive and communicative interventions. In E. M. & M. S. Bourgeois (Eds.), *Dementia: Person-centered assessment and intervention* (2nd ed., pp. 168–213). Taylor & Francis.

Hickey, E. M., Kinder, R., Khayum, B., Douglas, N. F., & Bourgeois, M. S. (2018). Setting the stage for person-centered care: Intervention principles and practical considerations. In E. M. & M. S. Bourgeois (Eds.), *Dementia: Person-centered assessment and intervention* (2nd ed., pp. 81–112). Taylor & Francis.

Kitwood, T. (1997). On being a person. In D. Brooker (Ed.), *Dementia reconsidered, revisited: The person still comes first* (2nd ed., pp. 6–23). Open university Press.

Mahendra, N., Fremont, K., & Dionne, E. (2013). Teaching future providers about dementia: The impact of service learning. *Seminars in Speech and Language, 34*(1), 5–17. doi:10.1055/s-0033–1337390

May, A. A., Dada, S., & Murray, J. (2019). Review of AAC interventions in persons with dementia. *International Journal of Language and Communication Disorders, 54*(6), 857–874. doi:10.1111/1460-6984.12491

McNaughton, D., Light, J., Beukelman, D. R., Klein, C., Nieder, D., & Nazareth, G. (2019). Building capacity in AAC : A person-centred approach to supporting participation by people with complex communication needs. *Augmentative and Alternative Communication, 1*–13. doi:10.1080/07434618.2018.1556731

Murphy, J., & Gray, C. M., & Cox, S. (2013). *Communication and dementia*. www.talkingmats. com/wp-content/uploads/2013/09/Dementia-and-Effectiveness-of-Talking-Mats-full-report1.pdf

Murphy, J., Gray, C. M., van Achterberg, T., Wyke, S., & Cox, S. (2010). The effectiveness of the Talking Mats framework in helping people with dementia to express their views on well-being. *Dementia, 9*(4), 454–472. doi:10.1177/1471301210381776

Nasreddine, Z. S., Phillips, N. A., Bédirian, V., Charbonneau, S., Whitehead, V., Collin, I., . . . Chertkow, H. (2005). The Montreal cognitive assessment, MoCA: A brief screening tool for mild cognitive impairment. *Journal of the American Geriatrics Society, 53*(4), 695–699. doi:10.1111/j.1532-5415.2005.53221.x

Riley, D. S., Barber, M. S., Kienle, G. S., Aronson, J. K., von Schoen-Angerer, T., Tugwell, P., . . . Gagnier, J. J. (2017, May). CARE guidelines for case reports: Explanation and elaboration document. *Journal of Clinical Epidemiology, 89*, 218–235. doi:10.1016/j.jclinepi.2017.04.026

Sackett, D. L., Rosenberg, W. M. C., Gray, M. J., Haynes, B. R., & Richardson, S. W. (1996). Evidence based medicine: What is it and what it isn't. *British Medical Journal, 312*(7023), 71–72. doi:10.1115/1.2899246

Schlosser, R. W., & Raghavendra, P. (2004). Evidence-based practice in augmentative and alternative communication. *Augmentative and Alternative Communication, 20*(1), 1–21. doi:10.1080/07434610310001621083

Williams, K. N., Kemper, S., & Hummert, M. L. (2003). Improving nursing home communication: An intervention to reduce elderspeak. *Gerontologist, 43*(2), 242–247. doi:10.1093/geront/43.2.242

World Health Organization (WHO). (2001). *International classification of functioning, disability and health: ICF*. WHO.

World Health Organization (WHO). (2017). *Dementia: Global action plan 2012–2025*. Retrieved, December 10, 2018, from www.Who.Int/Mental_Health/Neurology/Dementia/Action_Plan_2017_2025/En/

Index

Page numbers in *italics* indicate figures; page numbers in **bold** indicate tables.

Printed in the United States
by Baker & Taylor Publisher Services